MW00612681

Cover and line drawings by John Hughes
Line drawing editing and polishing by Mark Potter
Photographs by Meghan Eckman

Table of Contents

Acknowledgements

This book constitutes thirty years of hard work, research, and creativity. Many deserve mention for its completion and various features. I'm indebted to my friend and first real student John Dokken for holding steady with me for twenty-five years. Dr. Tyvin Rich merits special mention for contributing a preface and for helping to shape and continuously support the unconventional medical ideas contained in the book. Dr. Steven Pasternak also has provided invaluable assistance and input, and Professor Jeremey Tuttle did me a huge favor by reading and correcting early drafts of the manuscript. Mark Bernardino, Bill Smyth, and Doak Finch opened the door to greater credibility by giving my program a shot with the University of Virginia swim team, and for that I am forever grateful. My thanks also go to David Gerdt, Martin Baruch, Augie Busch, Professor Ann Gill Taylor, Terri Yost, Peggy Wright, Dr. Thomas Braciale, Professor Paul W. Ewald, Dr. Phillip Kuo, and Dr. Donald R. Fowler for working with me in the past to move the information forward into clearer light. I'm also grateful to Professor Lu Shaojun, Professor Xu Weijun, and Wang Zhenhua of the Beijing Wushu Institute for sharing their wisdom, and to Phil Midland for continuing to keep me connected with China and the bigger picture.

I also thank John Hughes for creating the cover art and for helping to articulate many of the book's core illustrations of the autonomic cardiovascular and immune system functions described in the text. Mark Potter has my deepest gratitude for completing and perfecting all the book's illustrations, which serve as a kind of vocabulary for Autonomic Intelligence.

Finally, I dedicate this book to my four sons Steve, Will, Luke, and Eryk, and to my wife Ania, who has stood by me during many long years of hardship and setback.

"So it is that whenever Heaven invests a person with great responsibilities, it first tries his resolve, exhausts his muscles and bones, starves his body, leaves him destitute, and confounds his every endeavor. In this way his patience and endurance are developed, and his weaknesses are overcome. We change and grow only when we make mistakes. We realize what to do only when we work through worry and confusion. And we gain people's trust and understanding only when our inner thoughts are revealed clearly in our faces and words." Mencius, 372-289 BC

Acronyms (in order of appearance)

A^uI = Autonomic Intelligence

RE = Reflective Exercise

RfR = Reflective Response

TBI = traumatic brain injury

AI = artificial intelligence

TCM = Traditional Chinese Medicine

ECG = electrocardiograph

HRV = heart rate variability

IR = inflammatory reflex

MRI = magnetic resonance imaging

HPE = Hawthorne-Placebo Effect

BPV = blood pressure variability

ENS = enteric nervous system

HEP = heart evoked potential

URI = upper respiratory infection

m-TBI = mild traumatic brain injury

CSF = cerebrospinal fluid

HMP = Human Microbiome Project

BWI= Beijing Wushu Institute

CNQI = China National Qigong Institute

CQA = Chinese Qigong Association

Chinese Terms (in order of appearance)

Fa gong—pronounced "Fah-goong": projected skill.

Nei Gong—pronounced "Nay-goong": internal skill.

Qigong—pronounced "Chee-goong": traditional Chinese mind-body exercise reputed to be at least 4,000 years old, sometimes spelled "Chi Kung" in the West.

Taiji or *Taijiquan*—pronounced "Tie-Gee" or "Tie-Gee-Chwan": slow-motion Chinese martial art, popularly known in the West as Tai Chi or T'ai Chi Ch'uan.

Wai Gong—pronounced "Why-goong": external skill.

Zi fa dong—pronounced "Zeh Fah Doong": automatic or trance movement.

Preface

As a practicing radiation oncologist for the last thirty-five years, I have always been interested in finding ways to improve the treatment for cancer patients. Several years ago I began to devote more attention to the causes of cancer patient's symptoms and to explore approaches to increasing the quality of life of those who suffer. Among these approaches, I gave special consideration to Traditional Chinese Medicine (TCM), in which I had always had an interest since my formative years in medical school. This interest, along with my growing focus on cancer symptomology, eventually led me to become medically certified in acupuncture.

Now my career allows me to combine both Western and Eastern philosophies into new logical approaches to further understand the nature of disease, especially with regard to cancer. TCM, like India's centuries-old medical system, describes all disease, including cancer, in terms of recognizable holistic patterns of "energy" imbalance. Remarkably, interventions based on these systems alleviate suffering in humans—the one and only goal, many times, the patient and their doctor hope to achieve. Western doctors and medical researchers attribute these helpful effects to tangible and intangible influences of the mind on the body's systems, with an unfortunate overemphasis on the intangible mind-body connection known as the "Placebo Effect." This dismissal overlooks the potential cause of a deeper, measurable mind-body connection, in particular the autonomic nervous system and its profound effects on health. Consequently, Western medicine has not invested much time and effort in careful investigations into the autonomic dimensions of some Far Eastern medical therapies.

A couple of years before I became interested in acupuncture certification, I met and began collaborating with John Alton, who in this book brings a strong argument for looking at the autonomic dimension in evaluating and shoring up health. He premises his argument on the concept of "Autonomic Intelligence," defined as the ability to build health through understanding and using the autonomic nervous system. This concept is helpful because it reconciles some of the apparent conflict between Western and Far Eastern definitions of the causes of good and poor health.

The book also describes a novel mind-body routine called "Reflective Exercise," which John distilled from the Chinese practice of Qigong. Reflective Exercise fits into a growing body of literature that explains the psycho-physiologic basis of meditation and adds to this understanding by examining the role of the autonomic nervous system in new ways. Although effects of mental stillness, breathing, and concentration have been well documented, the work John and I have done has produced new evidence, based on the study of heart rate variability, that immune wellness can be harvested by practicing Reflective Exercise. John calls this remarkable health effect the "Reflective Response," a cardiovascular sensation that moves from the lower abdomen into the head, measured as an instantaneous change in heart rate variability that prior research has shown is associated with a robust immune system.

The Reflective Response is probably a heretofore unknown type of "interoception," the documented ability to sense biological systems in real time. Interoceptive sensitivity likely varies from person to person, but Reflective Exercise and its hallmark Reflective Response may offer for many a means not only of building health, but also of targeting and treating health problems that stem from inflammation, the biological mechanism involved in virtually all known chronic diseases, including cancer.

The book also poses a credible theory of how Reflective Exercise creates the Reflective Response and builds upon both research and striking anecdotal evidence to offer stirring possibilities of individual control over biological systems long presumed to be out the conscious mind's reach. Some of these propositions remain to be tested, but they point the way to potentially revolutionary lines of inquiry.

As a medical scientist and physician devoted to the profession, I am committed to helping John continue to study and build on what we have observed thus far. It is my sincere hope that the ideas put forth in this book, foreign to conventional medicine up to now, can be better understood and applied to the benefit of humankind.

Tyvin A. Rich, MD, FACR

Professor Emeritus, Department of Radiation Oncology

The University of Virginia School of Medicine

Introduction

We live in an age where technology appears to have made most things more convenient and less expensive. One big exception to this rule is health care. Genomic and molecular analysis, imaging machines, electronic records, and high-tech procedures add to rather than reduce costs for health care. This trend has been underway since the 1980's and shows no signs of stopping, despite rosy predictions made by supporters of the Affordable Care Act, or Obamacare. In a 2014 presentation to a room packed with economists and healthcare specialists, Amitabh Chandra, director of Health Policy Research at Harvard's Kennedy School of Government, quoted an optimistic *New York Times* article that predicted sunny skies on curbing healthcare costs. Written in 1993, the article was referring to Clinton-era managed care, now roundly disparaged as a failure. Chandra was calling attention to the common approach to cost-cutting taken by both managed care and Obamacare: reduce bureaucratic waste. But he went on to point out that the real driver of healthcare expenses is medicine's continued love affair with costly high-tech treatments that often turn out to be no more effective than older, cheaper ones. What keeps this love affair going is that too many healthcare consumers are willing to pay for the newer, more expensive, dubious, high-tech treatments. This creates a vicious cost cycle that appears to have no end.

To its credit, Obamacare aims to break the cycle in the case of Medicare by paying only for therapies that produce good results. Though focused on the right problem, this solution has to answer two questions: how to define "good results" fairly and how to keep track of patients? The answers to both questions inevitably lead to more bureaucracy. Panels of experts will have to be convened to hammer out definitions of "good results" for a staggering number of diseases and treatments with different therapeutic time frames. New therapies, especially the expensive molecular ones, will require separate standards of evaluation. The panels will have to draft guidelines that will then have to be implemented, monitored, and enforced, all of which will produce a new bureaucratic layer of "health care" that someone will have to pay for, perpetuating the cycle of rising costs.

This book offers a different tactic in helping to break the cycle. It empowers readers with knowledge that gives them better control over the biological systems that determine health and illness. This empowering knowledge is called *Autonomic Intelligence* (*A^{u}I*), the capacity to regulate health through the autonomic nervous system, the biological bridge between mind and body, buried at the base of the brain and wired into the spinal cord and network of nerves riddling the flesh. Ordinarily, this mind-body connector acts invisibly, responding to the simplest movements and thoughts by revving the heart and pumping hormone-and-enzyme-enriched blood to every corner of the body as it plows through the energetic swales of the day. Enhancing A^uI increases knowledge of and control over the autonomic response not only to our immediate choices and actions, but also to perhaps the greatest demand life makes on us, the struggle to avoid short- and long-term illness.

Enhanced A^uI offers three advantages in this cradle-to-grave struggle. First, it provides select knowledge extracted from conventional medicine and biotechnology to explain the workings of the autonomic nervous system. Second, it clarifies known methods of promoting beneficial autonomic function and resilient good health. And third, it presents a method that has the radical effect of transforming the autonomic nervous system into a sensory organ, effectively opening a two-way communication channel between consciousness and two crucial biological processes the autonomic nervous system regulates: the cardiovascular and immune systems. The method is called *Reflective Exercise* (RE), and its transformative effect on the autonomic nervous system the *Reflective Response* (RfR). Experiencing the RfR over time leads to the development of the *pulsatile self*, a fusion of consciousness and the ability to sense and control the autonomic cardiovascular and immune systems.

Over the past ten years, studies conducted at the University of Virginia on the effects of RE and the RfR support the claim that the RfR constitutes healthy autonomic regulation of both the cardiovascular and immune systems. But for over twenty-seven years, over two thousand people have experienced its benefits. Most were average people with routine health concerns, but some were exceptional with exceptional problems that make a strong case for greater A^uI. Collegiate swimmers learned to use the RfR to self-treat injuries and respiratory diseases that plague them throughout their training and competitive season. Military veterans with traumatic brain injury (TBI) used it to manage crippling headaches and regain strength and function in enfeebled limbs. Individuals with mysterious chronic diseases that cause ongoing pain, fatigue, and cognitive dysfunction recovered a sense of normalcy with it. One woman diagnosed with terminal metastatic breast cancer was able to kill all the tumor sites in her body. Another man reversed coronary artery disease that doctors assured would end his life prematurely. These exceptional cases suggest that a common process connects mild and serious disease in terms of symptoms and recovery. Preponderant evidence points to the autonomic nervous system as the driver of this connection.

If the autonomic nervous system sits at the center of our general response to disease and injury, then the enhanced $A^u I$ provided by the RfR may extend into more obscure but important corners of the body's biology that recently have gotten a lot of attention. The microbiome—the body's inherent germ colony, located primarily in the gut—has been shown to exert considerable influence over autonomic function through chemical messages. The RfR may prove to be an effective method for managing those chemical messages, which can affect such basic drives as hunger and anxiety, both of which can lead to eating disorders and substance abuse and may be remotely causing serious diseases, such as heart disease, cancer, and diabetes. The RfR also may provide control over other autonomic health-regulating functions, such as eliminating enfeebled cells and stimulating the production of new tissues. For these possibilities to come about, the RfR must be experienced consistently over time, leading to the development of the pulsatile self, which conceivably could add decades of good health. The pulsatile self could make sixty the new forty.

By equipping readers with the background to understand $A^u I$ in general and with a method to make the leap to the greater $A^u I$ of the pulsatile self, this book has the potential to transfer to healthcare consumers some of the power held exclusively by an elite medical profession that does great work when treating advanced diseases with expensive procedures and drugs, but has failed to provide consistent and effective health-enhancing methods beyond advice on hand washing and obvious lifestyle choices, such as eating properly, getting enough sleep, exercising regularly, and learning to relax. Discovering the pulsatile self opens a pathway to better understand how to maintain health and avoid disease, and thus surpasses by good measure the current alternatives.

Part 1
A"I Fundamentals

Chapter 1
The Spiral of External Solutions versus Autonomic Intelligence

Early earth- and waterworks civilizations were the first to increase the supply and delivery of food, shelter, clothing, and other goods and services by altering the physical and social environment. This primordial tactic of manipulating the external environment to solve human problems uplifted civilization in Europe around the 16th century and since then has soared ever upward on the wings of one success after another, intensifying faith that it is the only way to go and at the same time fostering impatience to think things through. As a result, enormous amounts of human and financial capital have flowed toward engineering and technology solutions that generate unseen or underestimated troubles that demand new engineering and technical solutions. In time, the external tweaks that meet the demand lead to related or new problems that require more tweaks or entirely new technologies, which in turn consume more human and financial capital, thus creating an ever-expanding spiral of problem-causing solutions.

Examples in the 20th century abound. Single-crop and pesticide-intensive agriculture greatly increased grain production but ended up bolstering the grain-predatory insect population and poisoning the ecosystem, forcing a continual cascade of damage-control and restorative measures. The Army Corp of Engineers reconstructed the Mississippi River so that barges of grain and other goods could navigate more rapidly down to the Gulf of Mexico, but the changes wrought in the landscape caused massive flooding, which necessitated further civil engineering. Most recently, hydraulic fracturing, or fracking, introduced a new way to extract natural gas from underground by opening up subterranean seams with high velocity streams of water. Fracking increased American energy supplies to the point that it freed the country from dependence on Middle Eastern petroleum and caused the price of gasoline to plummet. But it also has side effects, including chemical contamination of the local water table and seismic instability, problems that supporters of fracking either deny or admit with the caveat that the damage is insignificant and eventually will drive the industry to search for remedies through "new technologies."

In fact, "dirty energies" such as oil, gas, and coal can take credit for much of the progress from the late-19th through the 20th century and the blame for the slowly developing global problem of climate change. Green energy is supposed to redress that problem. Self-driving electric cars promise to eliminate the collective damages inflicted by the single-driver internal-combustion car. Colonizing Mars carries the external-solution focus to its logical extreme by extending and redrawing the boundaries of the external map to create, if nothing else, excitement and hope that somehow the good times will keep rolling. Whether these solutions will have harmful effects downstream that will require more reengineering remains to be seen, but the chances are likely. Mars colonization certainly invites the imagination to consider a number of what-could-go-wrong sci-fi nightmares, such as the possibility of encountering and bringing back microbial life with evolutionary properties we are not prepared to deal with. Artificial intelligence (AI) may constitute the King Kong of external problem-causing solutions. Voices arguing for and against it are equally loud. The pros see AI as the key to a utopian dream, while the cons, including Stephen Hawking, warn that AI will inevitably lead to human extinction.

Whatever the cost of the spiral of external engineering to solve problems, the immediate reward of thinking exclusively in external problem-solving terms has conditioned a reflex to look nowhere else. The money and prestige are too intoxicating. Consequently very smart government leaders, scientists, businesspeople, entrepreneurs, and engineers find it almost impossible to consider simpler, internal solutions hiding in plain sight.

This is especially the case with health problems, one of humanity's most distracting threats. Ironically, diseases such as influenza, measles, smallpox, tuberculosis, and malaria sprang from perhaps the greatest external solutions to the problem of hunger—agriculture and animal domestication—which developed without the foreknowledge of parasitic microbes. With the invention of the microscope, 19th-century European and American medical scientists were able to find what appeared to be exclusively external causes for these and many other diseases—germs—and their work led to the development of external solutions in the form of antibiotics and vaccines. These solutions proved incomplete because they overlooked the possibility that germs can evolve immunity to antibiotics and vaccines. This oversight led to drug-and-vaccine-resistant microbial strains, which have been met with more of the same: novel drugs that manipulate the microbial environment, a solution that has created an arms race with no end in sight.

Solving health problems through chemical engineering on the microscopic level also formed a template that guided subsequent investigations of the genome, which microbiologists cast as an inner environment that, like the external one, can be tweaked and reengineered to redress health problems. Today, the lion's share of human and financial capital spent in medical research is aimed at figuring out what genes cause disease, which genes promote health, and what molecules can be manufactured to turn off the bad genes and turn on the good.

This relentless, high-paying foray into the molecular and even atomic level of the biological environment has done to health science what investment banking did to law and business schools up until the 2008 financial meltdown. The money and prestige shout down competing arguments. In particular, the louder and richer molecular and atomic approach to health science starves investigations into self-care, rendering them hopelessly modest, disconnected, and at best damned with faint praise.

In comparison to the self-healing arguments that have emerged to date, Autonomic Intelligence (A^uI) is immodest. Its core proposal that health can be created and stockpiled through increased understanding of the autonomic nervous system's wave-like, or *pulsatile*, nature may strike some as exaggerated, but the proposal is supported by physical data drawn from known health-science parameters. This distinction is an important one because unlike the less certain professions of investment banking and business law, health science responds more readily to physical data. Health science also demands that ideas be grounded in cumulative findings that bear up under repeated testing. A^uI meets this demand by aggregating and connecting past and ongoing research that shows what self-care approaches can do, helping to construct a coherent narrative of health and illness as something more than stacks and combinations of microscopic elements subject to randomness and the highly-educated (and expensive) potions expert. A^uI presents health and illness in terms of identifiable holistic patterns of oscillation in the autonomic cardiovascular and immune systems. At an advanced level, A^uI makes the oscillations of the autonomic cardiovascular and immune systems a part of real-time experience, transforming the individual into a pulsatile being.

The Basis of the Pulsatile Self

In recent years, Western philosophers and psychologists have come to embrace the Buddhist notion that the "self" is an illusion, that what we would like to think of as a singular coherent mind is actually an aggregate of multiple selves comprised of sensory memories, feelings, impulses, and ideas that shift over time and changing circumstances.

However true this might be philosophically or psychologically, in biological terms there is one certainty underpinning who we are: the autonomic nervous system, the pulsing core reactor that animates and tends our flesh and blood. The autonomic nervous system has no race, country, culture, or creed. It speaks the single complex language of oscillation, a multivariate waveform made flesh. Every second, our insides speed up and slow down, expand and contract, flame on and cool off, but these fluctuations are not binary and perfectly sequential. Like waves on the surface of turbulent water, they overlap and conflict with one another, apparently chaotic. But when observed over time, patterns that can signify health and illness emerge from this apparent autonomic chaos. These waveforms show up in the rise and fall of our energy levels during the day. They determine when we wake, eat, carouse, and sleep. But they also occur more frequently within shorter blocks of time, especially in the cardiovascular and immune systems.

These more rapidly occurring oscillations in the cardiovascular and immune systems are the basis of pulsatile reality and are the building blocks of long-term sustainable health. Learning how to generate and maintain variance in cardiovascular and immune oscillations is the basis of A^uI. Learning to sense and enhance those oscillations leads to advanced A^uI.

The A^uI Spectrum

A^uI is best understood in terms of a spectrum with three levels. What these three levels have in common is that they regulate the autonomic cardiovascular and immune systems for both short- and long-term benefit. What makes them different is the extent to which each involves sensory control of the autonomic cardiovascular and immune systems, in other words, a closer, more detailed working relationship between consciousness and the autonomic cardiovascular and immune systems, the foundation of the pulsatile self.

Figure 1

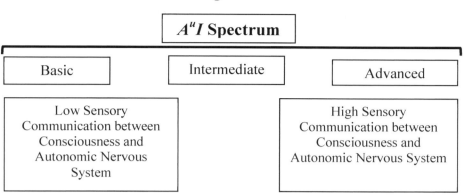

A^uI **Spectrum**

Basic	Intermediate	Advanced

| Low Sensory Communication between Consciousness and Autonomic Nervous System | | High Sensory Communication between Consciousness and Autonomic Nervous System |

Basic A^uI

At the left end of the A^uI spectrum, basic A^uI is characterized by learned voluntary acts that regulate the autonomic nervous system for both short- and long-term benefit. Resolving to not get upset over being stuck in traffic or a tedious business meeting as well as riding a bike to work or exercising more deliberately moves the autonomic nervous system from pure autoregulation and into the service of the conscious mind. Such voluntary acts provide only simple autonomic feedback, such as changes in heart rate, respiration, and temperature, but extensive research conducted over the past fifty years has demonstrated clearly the deferred benefits, not only on the healthy function of essential autonomic biological processes but also on the autonomic nervous system itself.

Basic A^uI is the product of over a million years of pre-human and human evolution and so tends to come naturally to most people. Any form of sustained movement draws upon our evolutionary aptitude for basic A^uI. Thus those who exercise regularly eventually acquire basic A^uI.

Intermediate A^uI

More discrete interactions between consciousness and autonomic nervous systems that require methods for sensing and smoothing out subtle, long-range autonomic perturbations constitute forms of intermediate A^uI. In the West, these methods entered the public square during the 1970's, but achieved more refined expression in the mid-to-late 1990's with the emergence of the Mindfulness and Emotional Intelligence movement.

Drawing on ancient "wisdom traditions" from the Far East and Western simplifications of those traditions, Mindfulness and Emotional Intelligence (from here on referred to collectively as Mindfulness) opened up the possibility of regulating the autonomic nervous system through simple meditative exercises and concepts. Intermediate A^uI may require a greater time investment in learning than do most forms of basic A^uI, especially if the intermediate methods and ideas are discovered later in life (which is largely the case for most Westerners). But once learned, intermediate A^uI like Mindfulness can help increase sensory awareness and control over autonomic biological processes through breath and attention to specific autonomic biological signals such as heart rate or more vague impressions such as levels of anxiety or lack thereof. Intermediate A^uI can disarm hidden emotional problems and disturbances that chronically destabilize the autonomic nervous system. In addition to Mindfulness, forms of cognitive-behavioral therapy, wherein an individual learns to identify, challenge, and disrupt impulsive and harmful behavior and thought patterns, qualify as intermediate A^uI. Furthermore, methods that fall into the category of intermediate A^uI have been shown to physically grow parts of the brain responsible for regulating emotion in much the same way lifting weights increases muscle mass.

Over the past twenty or so years, respected medical professionals have amassed a substantial body of research that shows the healthy effects of both basic and intermediate A^uI. While the beneficial effects of basic A^uI appear to be pretty self-evident, recent studies have shown that conventional cardiovascular exercise has a more profound impact than was previously thought. It can promote healthy changes in the genome (Zierth, et al).

Less self-evident is the proposition that an intermediate A^uI approach like Mindfulness could do the same, but the case has been made. Mindfulness pioneers Dean Ornish and Herbert Benson have shown that several intermediate A^uI exercises penetrate down to the genomic level. Before-and-after genetic profiles of groups of people who underwent eight weeks of training in these Mindfulness exercises showed an activation of genes associated with health and a deactivation of genes associated with stress (Dusek, et al, Ornish, et al).

This evidence shows the top-down health effect of engaging in A^uI activities such as conventional exercise and Mindfulness. Looking into what goes on at the top—namely the autonomic cardiovascular and immune systems—reveals not only the simplicity and relatively ease of building basic and intermediate A^uI, but also the singular way they achieve results.

Advanced A^uI

Basic and intermediate A^uI promote healthy function of the autonomic cardiovascular and immune systems, but they lack the capacity to provide sensory, real-time control of those systems. This capacity leads to the pulsatile self, and to get there, you need advanced A^uI. Reflective Exercise (RE) is the method of acquiring advanced A^uI presented here. There are other ways to achieve advanced A^uI, but they are grounded in the traditional thought and rhetoric of their Far Eastern cultures of origin. This has frustrated scientific efforts to study claims and effects that seem incredible and therefore undermine the demonstrable good those original methods can do. RE avoids this problem by keeping the focus on autonomic cardiovascular and immune effects and by framing its features in terms of the A^uI spectrum.

Advanced A^uI builds off of valuable elements of basic and intermediate A^uI. Like basic and intermediate A^uI, advanced A^uI involves movement, breathing, and attention to the present, but it tweaks these features in highly specific and nuanced ways. Its unique component involves focusing the sense of touch inward, which in combination with the other components leads to the emergence of the Reflective Response (RfR), the means of sensing and controlling the pulsatile self. The most probable biological explanation for the RfR is that the autonomic cardiovascular and immune systems have been transformed into a single sensory organ.

Externality and A^uI

Historically, all the various forms of A^uI have fallen repeatedly into the trap of trying to explain and justify themselves in external terms, which kindles a tendency to manufacture imaginative or philosophically biased interpretations that can obscure or even falsify effects. This is as true of basic as it is of intermediate and advanced A^uI. The object lessons of running expert Jim Fixx or the competitive cyclist Lance Armstrong illustrate the limits at the basic end of the spectrum. Focused exclusively on external markers of performance, basic $A''I$ can turn from a health builder to a kind of disease that wreaks both physical and psychological harm to oneself and others. Countless recent and historical abuses by gurus of various Far Eastern wisdom traditions suggest that intermediate and advanced levels of $A''I$ also can go from good to bad. They can intoxicate with an exaggerated sense of power, leading to self-deification (as in the time-honored Far Eastern tradition of master worship) and delusions that one somehow has tapped into the farthest reaches of the external plane, where physical and spiritual reality blend in a kind of twilight zone.

Framing the causes and effects of $A''I$ in terms of the degree of involvement with the autonomic nervous system helps to reduce the kinds of problems that stem from forever looking exclusively outside for answers. It allows effects to be measured, verified, and explained, creating knowledge composed of scientifically interpreted sensation. The pulsatile self is not illusory. It can be sensed, marshaled against a health problem, and measured within the parameters of medical knowledge.

Chapter 2
The Pulsatile Leap

Advanced A^uI requires making a "pulsatile leap," a real-time, sensory experience of the pulsatile nature of the autonomic nervous system. I made my leap almost thirty years ago, on a late-October night in 1987 on the campus of Beijing University, one of the few places at that time where such an A^uI enhancement was widely possible (a story to be taken up later). I had ended up at Beijing University because I fit the profile of what the administration was looking for in a foreign English professor—young, enthusiastic, and unencumbered by a family—but my own motive in applying for a job there was to heal a wrist bone that had been broken and then re-broken and traumatized so many times through fitness and martial arts training that it was essentially "dead" (another part of the forthcoming story). My plan was to get the injury treated with first-class Traditional Chinese Medicine (TCM), in particular acupuncture or herbal therapy, which I had come to believe in after experiencing temporary pain relief from several treatments in the U.S. But on my first evaluation, the Beijing doctor informed me that acupuncture and herbal treatments were too weak to remedy such a serious problem. Instead, the doctor recommended that I learn a traditional Chinese exercise that combines slow movement, breathing techniques, and meditation in both standing and seated positions. As part of my martial arts training, I had practiced a form of this traditional exercise that certain circles in Taiwan, Hong Kong, and California regarded somewhat highly. It had enabled me to feel extraordinary sensations, such as a thermo-electromagnetic-like energy radiating between my palms when I aimed them at each other. But after over a year's practice, the best I could say about this sensation was that it was just a cool thing to feel. It had no apparent health benefits, and certainly did nothing for my broken wrist.

Skeptical of the doctor's advice, I nonetheless did as I was bid because he was so certain that I could benefit. For a little over a month, I trained daily with several master teachers, and each had his own take on what constituted the best approach. Finally I settled on working with the Beijing University martial arts coach, who for an additional fee agreed to toss in martial arts lessons once my wrist healed up.

Practicing Martial Arts in Beijing's Imperial Garden

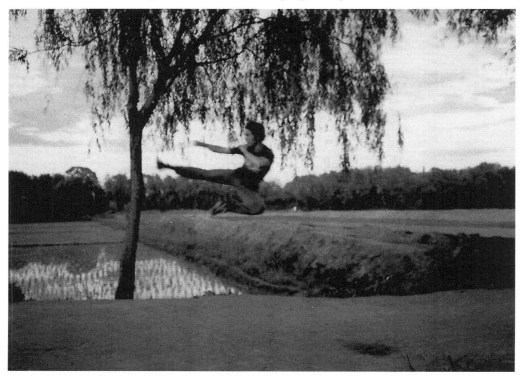

Aside from his expertise in martial arts, what attracted me to his approach was that one aspect of his routine involved feeling the thermo-electromagnetic sensation between the palms. But as with my experience back in the U.S., the magic appeared to have no effect my wrist, and after about a month of practicing his method, I started to lose what little faith I had. Not only was it time-consuming—two forty-five minute sessions daily—but several features seemed like foolish wastes of time. These included long stretches of lapsing into a ludicrous trance (which I never did) and an excruciating twenty minutes of meditating in an uncomfortable half-lotus position.

On the late-October night of my pulsatile leap, I sat in the annoying half-lotus on the floor of my apartment and entered the meditative phase of the routine with a bad attitude. The wind, howling off the Gobi desert, bumped and rattled the window in its ill-fitting frame like an angry spirit trying to get in. The noise reminded me of the building's creepy history as a former headquarters of Jiang Qing, Mao's famously ferocious widow, who twelve years earlier had reputedly imprisoned a young woman in my room and tortured her until she hung herself from one of the earthquake-retardant support cables that lined the walls near the ceiling. To top it off, a terrible upper respiratory infection made it hard to breathe, let alone manage the additional task of contracting and relaxing lower abdominal muscles in time with my breathing cycle. My head felt as though it were covered by a fishbowl of murky water. By all reckoning, it looked like I was in for a miserable, fruitless twenty minutes.

But then not more than five minutes in, a pulse sensation erupted in the center of my lower abdomen and shot straight up what felt like some sort of pathway into my head. My sinuses instantly cracked open as though I had inhaled decongestant steroids. Tears flowed and mucus ran. The pulse sensation rose from my lower abdomen to my head on inhalation and then fell back to its origin on exhalation. Each time the pulse ascended to my head, it seemed as though I was able to touch the source of the infection, which felt like a cyst. After hitting it with the pulse a few times, the cyst seemed to burst, and then it felt as though a swarm of tiny insects were scuttling across my face. Within less than a minute, the symptoms of the infection seemed to be gone. I spent the rest of the meditation relishing the smooth rise and fall of the pulse sensation and its seemingly miraculous healing effect, which so far as I knew no master teacher in the West had ever referenced. When I finished, I checked my face in the bathroom mirror and found a patch of reddish hives along either side of my nose and a pimple forming between my eyebrows.

In the months that followed, my devotion to the pulse sensation grew along with my ability to manipulate it. I started guiding the pulse sensation down into my "dead" wrist bone. X-rays taken five months later showed that the bone was restored, but I had all the proof I needed because I was back to doing wrist-stressing exercises, such as body presses on parallel bars and push-ups in both the prone and hand-stand positions.

Getting my right hand back sealed my dedication to the pulse sensation. I didn't know or care how, but I was determined to understand the pulse sensation and then help the rest of the world to understand it as well.

The twenty-plus years it would take to achieve that understanding was an evolutionary process toward the concept of A^uI, which replaces traditional Chinese explanations of both the exercise and the pulse sensation. Within the framework of A^uI, the pulse sensation goes from something mysterious and unscientific to something biological and *emergent*, the by-product of learning and practicing a simple routine with highly

Testing Healed Wrist Nine Months Later while Visiting Singapore

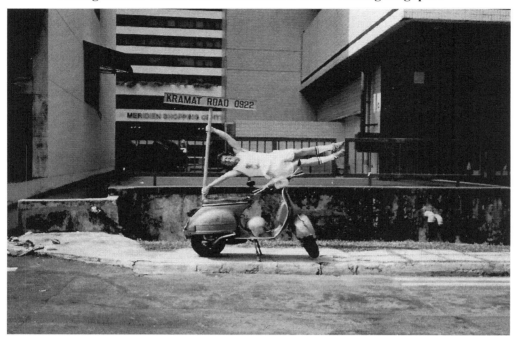

specific and nuanced features that lead to a plausible but extraordinary outcome: the pulsatile self.

One of these defining features involves sensing between the palms what appears to be thermo-electromagnetic-like energy. Though this energy sensation seems to come from the hands, its probable source is in the trunk and head of the body, where the autonomic nervous system ties the brain and vital organs into a complex oscillating system. This system produces electromagnetic, thermal, acoustic, and hydraulic forces that constantly flux throughout the baffles and channels of the head, chest, lower abdomen, and limbs. As these energies ricochet around inside the body, they produce "reflections," echo-like shifts that can be detected by medical devices. Given these verifiable conditions, it seems entirely plausible that if the body remained still for several minutes, the hands could sense some of these reflections in the air, especially in the chest area where the heart beat—a rhythmic process governed by the autonomic nervous system—generates some of the body's strongest reflections.

For this plausible reason, I decided to rebrand the routine *Reflective Exercise* (RE). It also works as a metaphor by suggesting that sensing the body's reflections to attain an inner picture resembles the way vision uses our reflection in a mirror to construct an outer identity. Calling the routine an *exercise* puts RE on a similar level with calisthenics, weightlifting, or swimming: a physical process that can be described in terms of movement, muscle groups, and breathing patterns. With this approach, RE becomes a form of auto-biofeedback that relies on the well-established principle of *neuroplasticity*, the capacity of the nervous system to form new pathways based on behavior and experience. Even better, the pulse sensation's emergence can be identified more objectively as a "Reflective Response" (RfR), a measurable autonomic effect with important health benefits. Thus far, all the objective and subjective data suggests that RE produces the RfR by transforming the autonomic nervous system into a sensory organ, which opens a fire-hose stream of real-time sensory data from the core regulator of biological life. Consciousness ordinarily

Illustration 1: The Reflective Response (RfR)

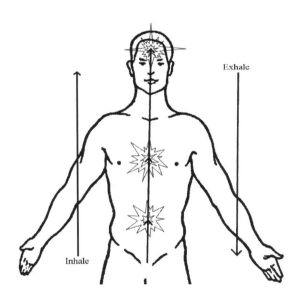

screens out most autonomic feedback. The RfR not only opens up some of that crucial real-time information, but also becomes a means of regulating the body's constantly fluctuating internal biology. This new information and ability constitute an advanced form of $A''I$ that makes ordinary reality *pulsatile*.

Some of the strongest support for these claims comes from four studies conducted at the University of Virginia that link the RfR to immune system balance and an important cardiovascular reflection that is widely accepted as a gauge of autonomic function. These studies and other evidence strengthen the hypothesis that the RfR is an emergent, neuroplastic pathway to sensing and regulating the autonomic nervous system. But they also place the RfR along the $A^u I$ spectrum that includes conventional exercise and popular meditative practices. The difference is that the RfR develops the pulsatile self by turning the autonomic nervous system into a sensory organ that allows for voluntary, real-time management of autoregulated biology. Thus the RfR may turn out to be the greatest, least known, and most poorly understood healing effect the world has ever seen.

Chapter 3
The Self as Waveform

The importance of the autonomic nervous system to overall health is indisputable. It interpenetrates the body's systems and constantly adjusts them in response to every movement or brow-furrowing thought. When the autonomic nervous system is in good shape, health endures. When the autonomic nervous system fatigues, disease and decrepitude follow. To keep the autonomic nervous system in good working order, it needs to be activated. In fact, autonomic non-use (and abuse) may be a primary cause of biological degradation over time. Thus, the first step in using A^uI to sustain health is to acquire a working understanding of the autonomic nervous system as the basis for the pulsatile self.

Autonomic Nervous System Anatomy

After reading this section, examine your own body in the mirror and imagine the key biological features discussed here. This will help you become more aware of the physical causes of the pulsatile nature of advanced A^uI.

The center of the autonomic nervous system resides deep within a region known as the brain stem. To locate this region, look in a mirror at your own face between your upper lip and eyebrows, and then imagine that you can see the diagram below inside this space toward the middle of your head. This is the rough location of brain central for the autonomic nervous system.

From this central location a network of nerve fibers fans out into the head, down

Illustration 2: The Brain Stem and Body Location of the Autonomic Nervous System

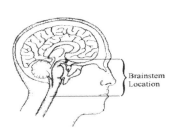
Brainstem Location

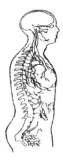

into the neck, chest, and lower abdomen. These fibers also join the densely packed cable of nerves running down the center of the spine, from where they exit and extend out into the trunk, pelvis, and the major organ systems.

Though the autonomic nervous system feeds into every visceral organ and marbles each tissue layer, the two aspects of the body most central to the pulsatile self are the cardiovascular and immune systems. The autonomic nervous system makes these two systems pulsatile by constantly driving them back and forth between three extremes: speeding up, constricting, and heating up versus slowing down, relaxing, and cooling off.

Figure 2

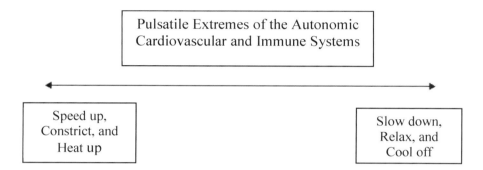

The Autonomic Cardiovascular System

The heart is the body's most immediately pulsatile organ, and it drives the cardiovascular system, which consists of a profusion of elastic arteries, joined to a sister network of veins (also elastic but less so than arteries) through which blood constantly circulates. The beating heart has four chambers and its own intrinsic oscillator called the sino-atrial node, a chemical battery of tissue that sets off a charge, causing the chambers to contract in a rapid sequence.

The top two chambers squeeze blood into the bottom two chambers, but the right and left side bottom chambers send blood to different places for different purposes. The bottom right chamber receives depleted blood from the top right chamber and then propels it into the lungs where the blood is oxygenated and returned through the pulmonary veins to the upper chamber on the left, which shoots its payload to the bottom left chamber from where the oxygenated blood gets ejected up into the aorta. This process takes less than one second for a normal heart. From the aorta, nutrient- and oxygen-enriched blood spreads

31

through arteries from the torso to the extremities. Once that job is done, veins return depleted blood for reenergizing through the organs and finally back to the heart and lungs for reinjection.

Illustration 3: The Cardiovascular System

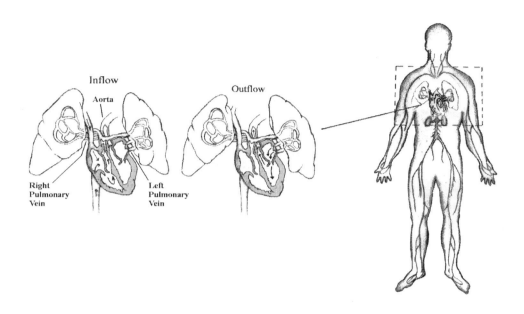

Second in importance to the heart is the aorta, the thickest, most voluminous, and most elastic blood vessel in the body. It emerges from the top side of the heart, bends sharply to the left, and forms an arch that feeds into a column that descends into the abdomen. From there, the aorta narrows and then branches in the pelvis into smaller arteries that project down into the legs.

Illustration 4: The Heart and Aortic Arch

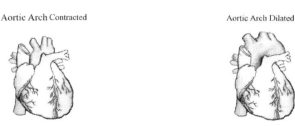

At the top, just above the arch, the aorta forms three smaller vessels that branch into the shoulders and neck. This arch formation absorbs and diminishes some of the force created by the blood load ejected at high velocity from the heart. The remarkable elasticity of the vessel helps to keep it from rupturing. Upon receiving a blood payload, it expands like a balloon and then squeezes back to its pre-expanded proportion, in the process driving blood into the other arterial branches.

Autonomic Cardiovascular Hydraulics

The cardiovascular system is hydraulic: an enclosed network of baffles and channels containing a pressurized fluid moved by a pump. The heart and the aortic arch constitute the pump, and their actions cause hydraulic pressure to vary. A fast heart puts more blood in the aortic arch, causing pressure to rise. Conversely a slow heart puts less blood in the arch and causes pressure to dip. To keep the system stable, a fast heart and increased aortic pressure must be countered at some point with a slower heart to prevent the aortic arch from bursting. Likewise, a slow heart needs to be sped up to keep the aortic arch from deflating and stagnating circulation. Thus a varying heart rate helps to maintain a hydraulic average or mean pressure in the central artery and throughout the cardiovascular system.

Through neuronal feeds to the heart, the aortic arch, and the carotid artery, autonomic central constantly works to keep mean pressure. It oscillates the speed of heart rates by syncing them with pressure changes in the arch. It does this by monitoring pressure through barometric and chemical sensory receptors in the arch and the carotid artery in the neck. The read autonomic central gets from these sensory receptors guides its use of a pair of switches that are embedded within the brain stem and are wired directly into the heart and into the barometric and chemical sensors of the aortic arch, and carotid artery. One switch increases the speed and force of heart contractions. The other slows and relaxes the heart. Unlike simple on-off switches, autonomic cardiovascular switches are *rheostats*, dials that can be turned up and down like the volume on a radio. They also can be turned simultaneously in either direction in an overlapping fashion. Autonomic central uses these rheostats in this non-linear fashion to adjust hydraulic pressure back toward its mean.

In medical parlance, the speed rheostat is called *sympathetic*; the relaxer is called *parasympathetic*. The heartbeat itself is self-driven, but when autonomic central turns up the sympathetic rheostat and turns down the parasympathetic, the speed and force of the beats increase so that heart contractions propel more blood into the aortic arch. To decrease the speed and force of the beats, autonomic central turns up the parasympathetic rheostat and turns down the sympathetic. The parasympathetic rheostat also feeds directly into the aortic arch through the largest physical feature of the autonomic nervous system: the *vagus nerve*. Though the vagus nerve is primarily part of the parasympathetic rheostat, it also shares a connection to the sympathetic rheostat. This connection between the vagus nerve and the sympathetic rheostat plays an important role in regulating the immune system, which will be discussed more fully later in this chapter.

Illustration 5: Autonomic Central's Sympathetic and Parasympathetic Rheostats and Pressure and Chemical Sensors in the Aortic Arch and Carotid Artery

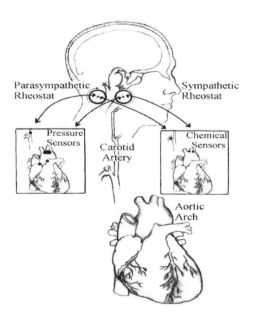

The influence of the autonomic rheostats manifests not in a single heartbeat, but over longer stretches of time. Changes in heart rate and blood pressure over these longer time intervals provide a window on autonomic central's continuous tuning of the sympathetic and parasympathetic rheostats to return pressure to its hydraulic mean, a necessary function for maintaining steady circulation of the blood throughout the cardiovascular system.

The Importance of Autonomic Cardiovascular Variance

In the late 19th and early 20th centuries, doctors began to comment that a varying pulse rate signified a healthy heart. With the development of electrocardiograph (ECG) technology, the ability to observe the autonomic cardiovascular system sharpened dramatically, and by the 1970's these observations stoked serious interest in the relationship between health and heart rate variability (HRV). After almost half a century of study and further technical improvements in ECG and other cardiovascular measurement technology, sufficient evidence has piled up in favor of HRV as a promisingly accurate, non-invasive way to observe patterns in the variable tunings of the sympathetic and parasympathetic rheostats. These patterns can reveal not only the autonomic nervous system's guiding role in regulating human biology, but also the pulsatile signatures of sickness and health.

The easiest to observe of the HRV regulatory patterns is the so-called *circadian cycle*, the twenty-four-hour rhythm of rest and activity that guides all biological life on Earth. During an active, alert state, heart rate and blood pressure tend to be high, indicating that the sympathetic rheostat is turned up and the parasympathetic rheostat has been turned down. In a resting state such as during sleep, heart rate and blood pressure drop, reversing the active settings of the rheostats. This circadian rhythm also determines similar patterns in other autoregulated bodily functions such as temperature (it rises when awake and drops when asleep) and metabolism (increased appetite while awake, satiation while asleep). Oscillations in the autonomic rheostats during the circadian cycle are assisted by *hormones*, molecules that cause cells to change or perform specific functions, produced in both the brain and the hormone-producing organs and tissues known as the *endocrine system*. Like their sympathetic and parasympathetic counterparts, hormones either speed and constrict or slow and relax the cardiovascular system.

The most famous of these hormones is adrenaline, which is produced by glands attached to the kidneys. Like the term *cardiovascular*, "adrenaline" is a piece of medical jargon that has entered the vernacular. Typically "adrenaline" is used to describe the

Illustration 6: The Circadian Cycle as a Waveform and Its Influence on the Autonomic Nervous System

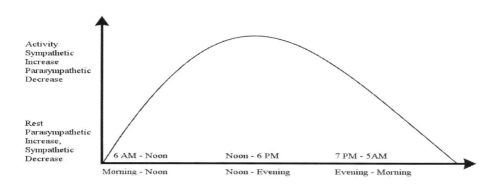

sympathetic "fight-or-flight" response, but this is true only when adrenaline release is high. When the body is at rest, adrenaline levels remain low and assist in parasympathetic relaxation. Within both the active and rest sides of the circadian cycle, however, heart rate and blood pressure vary, which means the sympathetic and parasympathetic rheostats are operating rhythmically within smaller time parameters. Medical researchers studying the rhythms of these smaller time spans have identified micro-patterns that predict both health and illness. These micro-fluctuations in the autonomic cardiovascular system also shape similar rhythmic patterns in the immune system, which handles both short- and long-term damage control.

Measuring HRV

The ECG (and other devices like it) captures the less-than-a-second electrical firing of the sino-atrial node and visually represents it as a three-part wave that consists of two small undulations on either side of towering spike. This three-part wave represents a heartbeat, and the height of the spike represents the maximum of the sequence of electrical forces that cause the heart muscle to contract, defined by the symbol "μV. Using the ECG, HRV can be calculated by measuring the duration of the rests between heartbeats, or *inter-*

beat intervals (see Illustration 7), in milliseconds and then counting the inter-beat intervals plotted against time in seconds, minutes, or hours.

Illustration 7: ECG

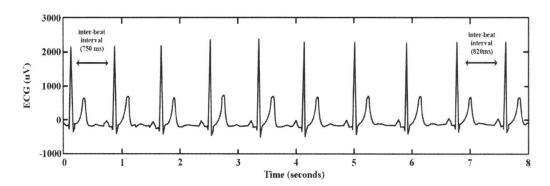

These calculations reveal a complex HRV waveform composed of smaller frequencies or wavelets. Between approximately one and five minutes, two kinds of smaller wavelets consistently emerge that have a strong correlation with autonomic function and health. These short-term wavelets are referred to as high and low frequency HRV. High frequency wavelets happen more often or with greater frequency. In a resting state, they begin and end on average every twelve to sixteen seconds, which comes to about

Illustration 8: High Frequency HRV Wavelet as Inter-beat Intervals in Milliseconds versus Time in Seconds

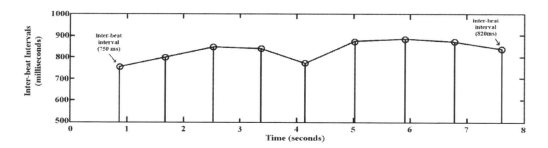

five complete oscillations every minute. Syncing the respiration cycle with this twelve-to-sixteen second timeframe increases high frequency HRV over time.

In contrast, low frequency wavelets occur less often (approximately every two minutes). Low frequency increases reflect autonomic processes that run deeper than respiratory patterns.

Variation or lack thereof in both low and high frequency HRV has been shown to correlate with health and illness respectively. Measures of robust high and low frequency HRV produce waves with steep peaks and deep valleys, and tend to indicate good health. Conversely, diminished peaks and valleys in both high and low HRV measurements are associated with sickness and vulnerability.

High Frequency HRV and Respiration

Respiration can increase high frequency HRV because the lungs connect to the heart and aorta in three ways. The first is purely hydraulic and seems on the surface counter-intuitive. When the lungs fill with air, the relative pressure inside the lungs is less than the pressure inside the pulmonary vein, which channels blood directly into the heart. The pressure difference causes the pulmonary vein to swell, which slows blood flow to the heart. Autonomic central reads this decrease in blood flow and dials up the sympathetic

Illustration 9: the Hydraulic and Parasympathetic Effects of Respiration

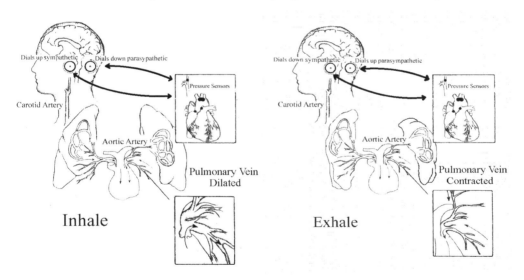

rheostat while dialing down the parasympathetic to speed the heart in an effort to compensate for the decreased blood flow that the heart can propel into the aorta, thus making for less internal aortic pressure. With the heart beating faster, the inter-beat intervals will decrease (see Illustration 10). Out-breaths reverse the hydraulic conditions. As the lungs deflate, the pressure difference between the inside of the lungs and the pulmonary vein diminishes, and the pulmonary vein squeezes its blood store into the heart.

Autonomic central responds to this increased blood flow by dialing down the sympathetic rheostat and dialing up the parasympathetic, decreasing heart speed to keep the aortic arch from over-expanding from increased pressure of greater blood flow. These modulations cause inter-beat intervals to increase (see Illustration 10).

The overall effect of this respiratory dynamic is that in-breaths tend to increase heart rate and decrease blood pressure and inter-beat intervals, while out-breaths decrease heart rate and increase blood pressure and inter-beat intervals.

Illustration 10: High Frequency HRV Graph of the Hydraulic and Parasympathetic Effects of Respiration

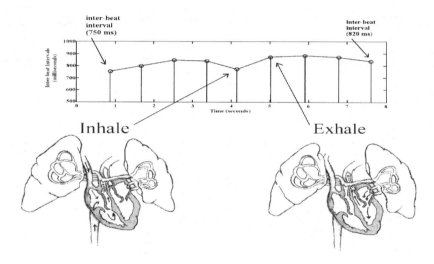

The second connection between the lungs and the heart and aorta is the vagus nerve, the Mac-daddy of the parasympathetic rheostat. This connection is similar to that of the vagal pressure sensors inside the aortic arch. When the lungs take in air and expand, similarly embedded vagal pressure sensors trigger a parasympathetic dial-up, which counters the hydraulic dynamics of the in-breath (heart rate speed-up and blood pressure dip). Conversely, out-breaths relax the pressure sensor, which dials the parasympathetic rheostat back down. These actions triggered by the vagal pressure sensors in the lungs run contrary to autonomic central's increased sympathetic action taken to handle the increased mechanical hydraulic pressure caused by the surge of blood from the pulmonary vein to the heart, but together they continually strive to restore the cardiovascular system to a stable state within a very short stretch of time.

The third way respiration affects HRV is through chemical sensors that sit just above the pressure sensors in the aortic arch (also, along with pressure sensors, in the carotid artery in the neck). These chemical sensors detect and communicate to autonomic central changes in the acid, oxygen, and carbon dioxide levels of the blood that fluctuate primarily because of respiration. When the lungs take in air, they extract oxygen from the gases that compose the air, and then exhale carbon dioxide and other waste gases. In addition to these respiratory changes, chemical levels also fluctuate because increases and

Illustration 11: Chemical Effects of Respiration on HRV

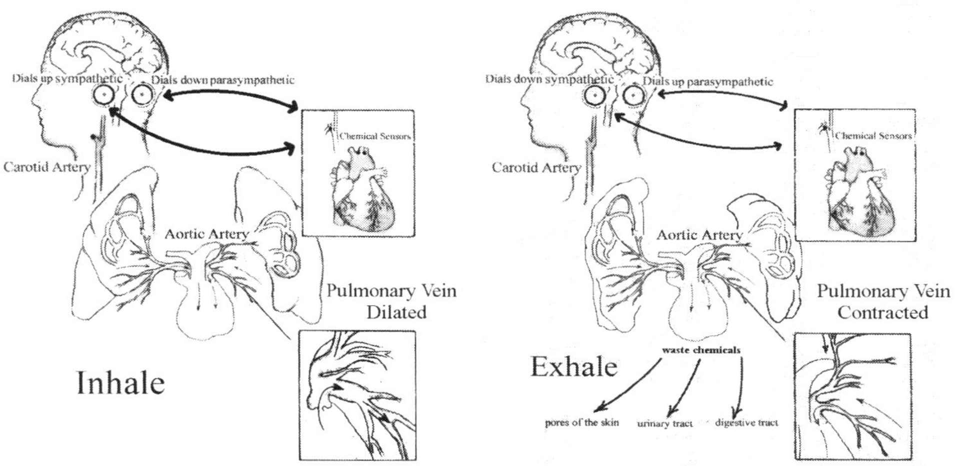

decreases in pressure cause the temperature of the blood to go up and down (another condition monitored by autonomic central). Increased pressure heats blood and thus can break apart the bonds holding molecules together, increasing waste such as carbon dioxide, which has to be routed out of the body. Guided by feedback from these chemical sensors, autonomic central also uses the sympathetic and parasympathetic rheostats to get rid of these waste chemicals through the pores of the skin and urinary and digestive systems.

Low Frequency HRV and Autonomic Balance

Circadian rhythms constitute the lowest frequency wavelets in HRV, but other low frequency wavelets emerge after about one hundred and twenty seconds of continuous ECG. These low frequency wavelets do not cohere with high frequency wavelets and thus respiration does not exclusively drive them. Over the past several years, the HRV research consensus is that these low frequencies in HRV indicate that autonomic central is trying to restore balance to cardiovascular rhythm and pressure by oscillating the sympathetic and parasympathetic rheostats. Growing evidence suggests that feedback and feed-forward loops between autonomic central and the vagal pressure sensors in the central arteries also could be behind this equalizing activity. This makes low frequency HRV a marker of the autonomic cardiovascular system's constant effort to evenly distribute hydraulic pressure.

Illustration 12: Low Frequency HRV Graph as a Measure of Autonomic Balance

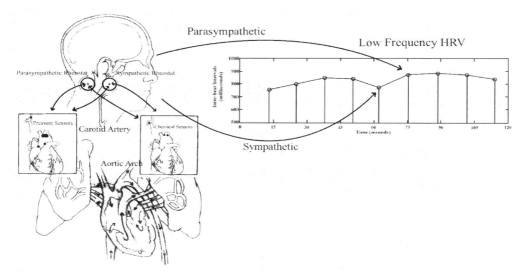

The HRV-Health Connection

In the past fifteen years, growing evidence suggests that HRV is a reliable marker of good and bad health. Studies involving large numbers of people have shown that ECG readings with increased HRV tend to indicate good health, while readings with decreased HRV tend to bode poorly. These investigations took place during the time researchers were finding that high levels of inflammation—a chemical reaction in the immune system—substantially contribute to the development of most chronic, lethal diseases, such as atherosclerosis, cancer, and diabetes. This led HRV researchers to study the relationship between HRV and inflammation, which turns out be an inverse one. In other words, increased HRV and low levels of inflammation tend to go together. The opposite is true of decreased HRV. The Cardia Study—the largest investigation to date—found a strong

41

inverse link between HRV and inflammation in more than seven hundred fifty people over a fifteen-year period (Sloan, et al.).

In parsing HRV further into high and low frequencies, arguments have begun to congeal around observations that increases in lower frequencies correlate with improved immune function. These findings show that autonomic cardiovascular and immune systems are deeply intertwined and are pulsatile in nature.

The Pulsatile Nature of the Autonomic Immune System

Like the autonomic cardiovascular system, the autonomic immune system is driven by the sympathetic and parasympathetic rheostats. But instead of speeding up and slowing down through constriction and relaxation, the rheostats act more like thermostats, making the immune system heat up and cool off.

Figure 3

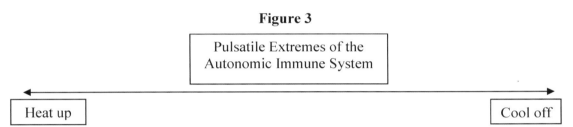

The sympathetic thermostat turns up and down the heat; the parasympathetic thermostat turns up and down the coolness. Like its cardiovascular counterpart, the autonomic immune system uses a feedback and feed-forward communications system, but unlike its cardiovascular counterpart, which manages hydraulic pressure through sensors embedded in the central and carotid arties, the immune system uses cellular agents to perform its job, which consists of detecting and dealing with infectious microbes, wear-and-tear, and blunt-force trauma. Once they find a problem, they signal autonomic central, which responds by dialing up and down the sympathetic and parasympathetic thermostats.

In this regard, the immune system's cellular agents resemble an ideal national guard, defending the homeland against invaders and repairing and restoring after foreign attacks and natural disasters. This guard is on constant alert, patrolling the body through its own network of channels called the *lymphatic system*, which like the cardiovascular system ramifies throughout the body. Fluid carrying the immune-system army fills lymphatic channels the way the blood suffuses cardiovascular vessels. But the lymphatic system has no pump like the heart to propel its contents. It relies instead on whole body activity and increases in blood pressure to provide that driving force. Some of that increased pressure reaches lymphatic channels through tiny capillaries that allow the immune-system army to go back and forth between the lymphatic and cardiovascular systems. But the biggest feed between the two is the *thoracic duct*, located on the left side of the neck, which dumps lymphatic fluid directly into the blood stream.

Illustration 13: the Lymphatic System's Connection to the Cardiovascular System

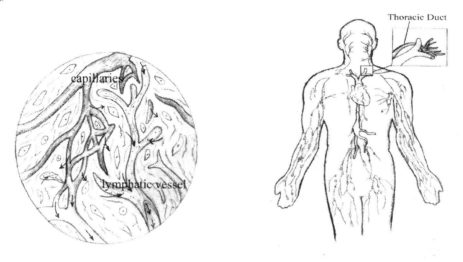

Broadly speaking, all cellular agents of the immune-system army are *lymphocytes* (white blood cells), but they vary according to size, shape, and function. Lymphocytes either circulate through the interconnecting corridors of the lymphatic and cardiovascular systems or garrison in way-station-like glands, the largest and most plentiful of which are in the gastrointestinal tract, otherwise known as the gut. The likely reason for this location is the vast number of microbes that dwell in the gut's lining, which frequently experiences micro-tears that spill germs into the bloodstream. Having the lion's share of the army in the gut is likely the result of evolutionary germ warfare stretching back over eons.

In the gut and elsewhere in the body, lymphocyte soldiers are in constant conflict and negotiation with microbial parasites and tagalongs, and, like all the body's cells, lymphocyte soldiers eventually tire, age, and begin to die. Younger lymphocyte soldiers detect and weed out these disabled veterans and signal for replacements that are formed mainly in the bone marrow and to a lesser extent in the lymph glands. The replacements go where they are needed, but most follow the historic migratory path to the glandular way stations in the gut.

If the cellular agents of the immune system are an army, then autonomic central is the army's central command, or in Pentagonese, AutCentCom. AutCentCom receives intelligence from the army and issues commands to it through both the sympathetic and parasympathetic thermostats. Generally speaking, the sympathetic thermostat sends and receives attack-molecular signals called *cytokines*, while the parasympathetic monitors and modulates aggressive action by producing stand-down cytokines. Attack cytokines incite *inflammation*, and thus are called *pro-inflammatory*. The stand-down cytokines dampen inflammation and are called *anti-inflammatory*. To sharpen the point even finer, think of cytokines equipping some lymphocyte soldiers with flame-throwers (pro-inflammation) and others with fire hoses (anti-inflammation).

AutCentCom uses the sympathetic and parasympathetic thermostats to balance the flame-throwers and fire-hosers as it does with pressure in the cardiovascular system. Its primary field commander is the vagus nerve, which wanders (*vagus* is Latin for "wander") down into the all the internal organs of the trunk and lower abdomen. Though it has important pressure sensory feeds into the aortic and carotid arteries, vagal nerve endings are most plentiful in the gut, where the majority of the lymphocyte army patrols and garrisons. These vagal gut fibers are the main place where inflammatory orders are given. But cytokine signals run both ways. The lymphocyte army patrolling the cardio-lymphatic corridors also provides intelligence to AutCentCom that shapes its orders.

When lymphocyte soldiers encounter damage or an invader, they flame on and corrode the problem. Local sympathetic nerve fibers detect the corrosion and signal the sympathetic arm of the vagus nerve, which informs AutCentCom, which then sends out an endocrine support team of anti-inflammatory hormones that assist in cooling off the attack process. Adrenaline and cortisol are the most well-known of these anti-inflammatory hormones.

Autonomic central uses the sympathetic and parasympathetic thermostats to maintain mean equilibrium between fire and water in the immune system the same way it uses them as rheostats to restore mean hydraulic pressure in the cardiovascular system. High blood pressure, a racing heart, and high levels of pro-inflammatory cytokines generate sickness symptoms, such as fever, aches, nausea, weakness, fatigue, dizziness, and general malaise. When pro-inflammatory levels go too high, the autonomic cardiovascular system and other autonomically regulated vital organs can fail. This is what happens in severe infectious conditions like septic shock.

AutCentCom fights off such catastrophes by telling the vagal field commander to begin replacing flame-throwers with fire hoses until order is restored. This autonomic-immune restorative process came to light in 2002 and has been labeled the *inflammatory reflex* (IR) (Tracey). This fairly new understanding of how the autonomic nervous system

Illustration 14: Flame-thrower and Fire-hoser Analogy of the IR

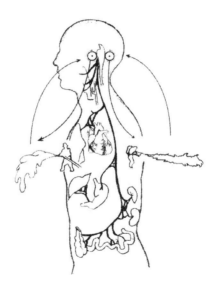

regulates immune responses has provided insight into mortal health problems that are associated with excess inflammation, such as heart disease, cancer, and diabetes, as well as non-lethal but chronically debilitating illnesses such as asthma, arthritis, and unknown-cause rheumatic diseases, formerly referred to as chronic fatigue and fibromyalgia. Medical scientists studying the role of the IR in chronic inflammatory disease are looking for molecular ways to restore pro- and anti-inflammatory balance.

But in a complex world where movement and constant interaction with both the macro-and micro-environment constantly destabilizes both the IR and the autonomic cardiovascular system, a genomic or chemistry lab may be the wrong place to look for a magic bullet. A simpler and more efficient solution may be to teach people to develop and enhance $A^u I$.

Chapter 4
The Unconventional Benefits of Basic A^uI

Most people do conventional exercise because they want to *look* physically fit. They measure their look by weight loss, muscle size, or improved performance, such as the ability to do more repetitions or run faster.

Looking more fit or winning some physical contest is immediate and superficially satisfying, but neither can match the health value of the deeper, hidden exercise effects on the autonomic cardiovascular and immune systems. Simply getting up out of a chair immediately affects the autonomic cardiovascular system. The leg muscles, some of the largest in the body, flex and squeeze veins and arteries and thus increase blood pressure in the periphery. The pressure sensors in the central artery read this increased pressure and transmit the information to autonomic central, which sets off a domino-like series of adjustments of heart rate and arterial diameter.

Prolonged movement maintains this cascade of effects and thus works and strengthens the autonomic nervous system the same way exercise works and strengthens muscle. In both cases, the benefits accrue downstream over time, but the autonomic effects will be harder to see than bigger biceps. Brisk walking and running achieve their good results by turning up the sympathetic rheostat and keeping it there, which forces compensatory tuning in the parasympathetic rheostat. These exercises accomplish this by making lower body muscles squeeze blood vessels so that peripheral pressure increases, especially in the veins, which then pushes blood in greater volume to the heart. Autonomic central responds to this increased blood flow by speeding the heart, which ejects its larger payload into the aorta, causing central pressure to skyrocket and body temperature to rise. Not for nothing are the legs referred to as a "second heart." To keep the cardiovascular engine from blowing, autonomic central dials up the parasympathetic rheostat, but the sympathetic rheostat remains dominant until the movement stops. If this goes on for twenty to thirty minutes—the generally prescribed time for cardiovascular exercises like brisk walking or running—the blood stream becomes saturated with both sympathetic and parasympathetic chemicals and hormones. Adrenaline is especially high, producing a "flight-or-fight" sympathetic effect conditioned into the autonomic cardiovascular system through eons of evolution. After the exercise is over, adrenaline

Illustration 15: Effects of Walking or Running on the Autonomic Rheostats

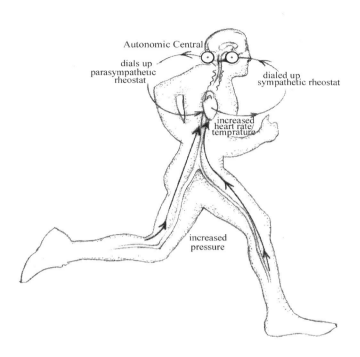

levels drop and can then assist its hormonal cousin cortisol not only in lowering blood pressure but also in hosing down the IR. Cooling down or taking a full-blown nap after brisk walking or running assists in parasympathetic correction.

Respiration: the Parasympathetic Counter-punch

Respiration during conventional exercise also assists in dialing up the parasympathetic rheostat to counter the sympathetic effects of exercise. It does this in two ways. The first is chemical; the second is mechanical. Both involve the pressure and chemical sensors in the aortic and carotid arteries.

Conventional exercise like running imposes a vigorous respiratory cycle that sends the at-rest chemical balance of the blood into chaos. The exchange between oxygen inflow and carbon dioxide outflow is also larger and more rapid. In-breaths supply fresh oxygen,

48

which provides the energy needed to maintain the heightened sympathetic response to

Illustration 16: The Role of Chemical Sensory Receptors in Vigorous Respiration

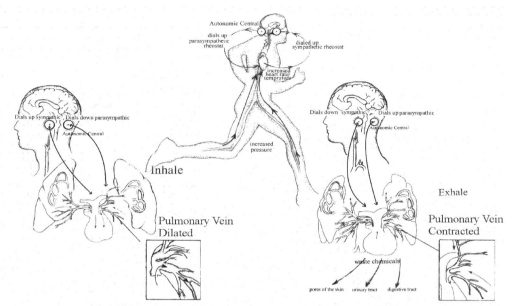

continued exercise. Out-breaths expel carbon dioxide and other noxious gases that promote sympathetic elevation. This carbon dioxide outflow is also larger and more rapid. This rapid gas exchange puts the arterial chemical sensors to work monitoring the blood's changing levels of oxygen, carbon dioxide, and acidity, signaling autonomic central to turn up the parasympathetic rheostat and turn down the sympathetic, which modulates heart rate and arterial diameter and opens the pores of the skin. These actions ventilate and cool body temperature to avoid excessive molecular breakdown in the blood.

The mechanical parasympathetic effects of respiration are more direct. Pressure sensors wired into the lungs and the barometric effects of respiration on the pulmonary vein trigger modulations in the autonomic rheostats. In-breaths simultaneously dial up the parasympathetic and the sympathetic, while out-breaths reverse the situation. While rapid exercise breathing forces the sympathetic and parasympathetic rheostats to oscillate in this way, its overall effect on autonomic central is to keep the cardiovascular system at an elevated sympathetic level.

In proper doses, the fixed autonomic relationship between breathing and the cardiovascular system can make any conventional exercise that coordinates breath to

Illustration 17: The Mechanical Effects of Exercise Respiration on the Autonomic Cardiovascular System

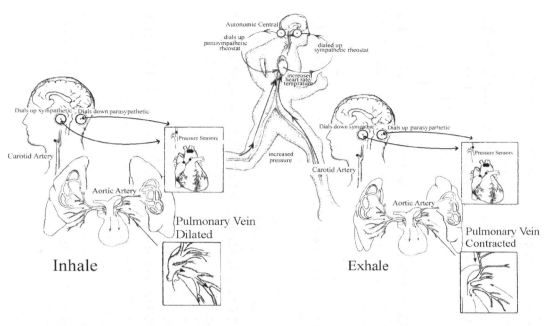

movement a form of basic $A''I$. Muscular exertion should be timed with out-breaths, such as when lifting a weight, hitting a ball with a bat or racket, throwing a punch or kick, or thrusting alternating handfuls of water past the body while swimming. Conversely, the muscles should relax on in-breaths. With sustained aerobic exercise like running or brisk walking, counting rhythmically so that the legs push harder on alternating intervals of out-breaths than on in-breaths similarly cultivates basic $A''I$. Coordinating breath to movement in these ways challenges and works the natural oscillations of the autonomic cardiovascular system.

By the same token, exercising with irregular breathing or over-exercising can destabilize and even harm the autonomic cardiovascular system. Studies on marathon runners, elite swimmers, and Navy SEALs show that after extremely vigorous exercise autonomic cardiovascular oscillations can become unhealthy. While healthy oscillations usually return during recovery from extreme exercise, the evidence suggests that the benefits of persistent extreme exercise eventually vanish and turn harmful.

The Effects of Conventional Exercise on HRV

Because conventional exercises like brisk walking and running force the autonomic nervous system to balance the pressure and chemical demands wrought by movement and vigorous breathing, it should not be surprising to see greater HRV in the resting ECG's of those who habitually exercise three to five times per week. Large and small studies confirm this effect. The greatest increases tend to be in the high frequency range. Beneficial increases in low frequency HRV show up in those below middle age, but tend to diminish after that. Thus, the HRV evidence suggests that enhanced respiration through movement is the main aspect of conventional exercise that bestows autonomic cardiovascular benefits (Sandercock).

Conventional Exercise and the IR

Since the cardiovascular and immune systems are autonomically connected, it seems logical that conventional exercise could work the IR through its autonomic connection. Multiple studies have confirmed this. More specifically, these studies establish a strong relationship between increased HRV and a relatively cool IR (Pinto). The IR's response to oscillations of sympathetic and parasympathetic thermostats provides an understanding of how this could happen. Conventional exercise likely increases levels of inflammatory cytokines for two reasons. First, any exercise that involves prolonged movement for twenty to thirty minutes will mildly traumatize musculoskeletal tissue, provoking the IR to remove damaged cells via the interplay between flame-throwers and fire-hosers. Second, the sympathetic dominance induced by twenty to thirty minutes of continuous exercise probably further excites the flame-throwing, pro-inflammatory side of the IR. To keep the pro-inflammatory increase in check, AutCentCom keeps tabs via the sympathetic connection to the vagal field commander, which issues stand-down orders and increases the number of fire-hosers, including massive anti-inflammatory hormonal support from cortisol, just as the autonomic cardiovascular system counters sympathetic overdrive with parasympathetic outflow. This anti-inflammatory correction succeeds only after exercise ends, when cool-downs or follow-on power naps can assist in restoring equilibrium between fire and water in the IR.

Illustration 18: The Effects of Conventional Exercise on the IR

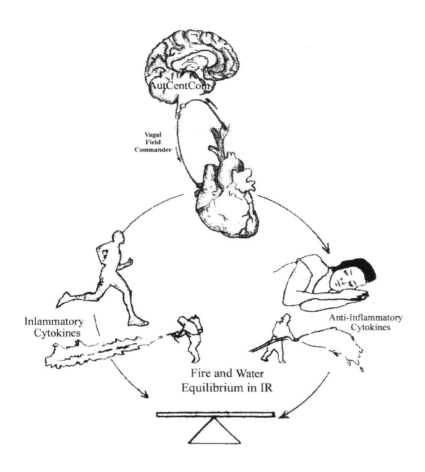

The Bottom Line of Basic A^uI: Move It or Lose It

Long periods of immobility can cause the autonomic cardiovascular and immune systems to diminish and waste away the same way muscles and bone dissipate as a result of inactivity. Simple conventional exercises such as brisk walking and running strengthen and tone the autonomic cardiovascular and immune systems by working them. As conventional exercise becomes a regular experience, the exerciser gets feedback in the form of an overall improved sense of wellbeing, a remote effect of autonomic health. Using known guidelines such as target blood pressure or heart rate measurements can also provide feedback. This serviceable information, along with the understanding that the overwhelming evidence that regular exercise is healthy, makes conventional exercise the easiest form of basic A^uI to acquire. All you have to do is carve out twenty to thirty minutes a day for sustained movement of some kind and the benefits begin to accrue. But the big payoff occurs in the long run, because a strong and well-toned autonomic nervous system provides the best protection from the vicissitudes of aging.

Notes on Diet and Sleep

Regular exercisers who don't eat and sleep properly will quickly lose whatever benefits their basic A^uI routines provide. Thus, regular exercise, diet, and sleep form a three-legged stool that constitutes basic A^uI. But whereas exercise incites heightened oscillation between sympathetic and parasympathetic outflows, healthy diet and sleep are mostly parasympathetic affairs. As such, they tend to dampen oscillation in cardiovascular and immune systems. Eating causes blood flow to increase in the gut to help promote digestion, which causes heart rate, blood pressure, and the IR to idle. Sleep has similar effects. During sleep, the vagus nerve—the strong right hand of the parasympathetic channel—becomes highly active, lowering heart rate and blood pressure and hosing down the inflammatory aftermath of the day.

Disturbances in both digestion and sleep are signs that healthy autonomic oscillation has been lost. Changing to a diet that dampens the sympathetic channel and organizing a rest-activity schedule closer to the Earth's natural light-dark cycle can restore healthy autonomic rhythms, but the results take time to accrue. Making time for conventional exercise four to five days a week can speed things along because exercise directly compels the autonomic cardiovascular and immune systems into proper rhythm.

A couple of simple rules of thumb in diet and sleep can help promote basic A^uI. First, eat a balanced diet rich in fiber (whole grains, fresh fruits, and fresh vegetables), protein, and fat. Dietary arguments are abundant and noisy, and they are attractive because, unlike conventional exercise, food is immediate, gratifying, and easily managed in the comfort of home, a place of parasympathetic peace, away from prying judgments. Diets are also highly susceptible to social distortions, shaped unconsciously by family, custom, and peers. But without adequate activity, no dietary approach will restore healthy rhythm in the autonomic cardiovascular and immune systems. From an A^uI perspective, an enjoyable diet that satisfies the "balanced" rule of thumb is a good starting point.

Sleep is at least as essential as diet for maintaining healthy levels of activity. Unless you have a rare "night owl" gene, which reverses the normal circadian cycle, a healthy rest-activity rhythm should approach Benjamin Franklin's "early to bed, early to rise" principle: wake up and move around when the sun is up and then decompress and sleep when darkness falls. Exercising vigorously during the day also can promote decent sleep.

These steps are simple, self-evident matters of will power and scheduling, but many resist. Some do so because they have either consciously or unconsciously subordinated their own health to other behaviors and activities. Others may feel that attempting to control health is futile, that chance overrules planning. These excuses fly in the face of medical facts that basic A^uI rests upon. Living by distraction and reliance on chance is more apt to produce health problems than taking the necessary steps to acquire basic A^uI.

Chapter 5
Intermediate A^uI and the Illusory Self

Some seemingly meditative practices, such as strenuous forms of yoga (Bikram and Hatha yoga, for example) and the apparently laconic martial art *Taiji* (Tai Chi), build basic A^uI the same way conventional exercise does: by regulating respiratory patterns and straining muscles to create pressure shifts in peripheral circulation, which forces autonomic central to work the overall autonomic cardiovascular and immune systems. But meditative methods like Mindfulness cultivate intermediate A^uI by tackling the illusory self, which, however fleeting and ephemeral in the grand scheme, can distort autonomic oscillations and degrade health even in those who appear to be fit. Ripped abs, bulging pecs, and flaring lats are no match for hidden anxieties that can lead to self-destructive behavior or a gradual loss of oscillation because of being stuck in perpetual sympathetic overdrive.

Intermediate A^uI methods such as Mindfulness diffuse sympathetic-driven stress by directing attention to details in the moment or by patiently coaxing out hidden anxiety so that it can be calmly observed and disarmed. In these ways, intermediate A^uI deflates the power of old psychological wounds and exposes false coping strategies that have become vicious cycles of fixed autonomic imbalance. Those caught in theses vicious cycles may so strongly identify with their coping strategies that they *become* the cycle. Intermediate A^uI dissipates the hold of the cycle by urging constant awareness of the present moment and the breath. Troubling thoughts or memories are encouraged to emerge where they can be observed without judgment. Somewhere in this process, a sense of release begins to occur, and an alternative perspective may appear to unfold organically. As this new perspective takes hold, anxiety lessens, conflict with others diminishes, a general sense of peace settles in. This change finds its most demonstrable effects in improved social relationships, which can strengthen the autonomic cardiovascular and immune systems. Less apparent but more profound is the possibility of enhancing brain anatomy. Using magnetic resonance imaging (MRI), researchers compared the brains of those who practiced eight weeks of Mindfulness with those of a control group that did nothing and found in the Mindfulness group significant increases in areas of the brain involved in learning, memory, and emotional regulation (Hölzel, et al).

Breath, Focus, and Compassion: the Tools of Intermediate A^uI

Healthy autonomic changes wrought by Mindfulness and other intermediate A^uI methods can be attributed largely to respiration, based on the same mechanisms described in conventional exercise. Intermediate A^uI respiratory methods lack the muscular strain that jacks up the sympathetic channel, and so tend to promote parasympathetic dominance. But like conventional exercise, they also promote healthy changes in HRV.

Effects of Intermediate A^uI Breathing Methods on High and Low Frequency HRV

Breathing patterns set up mechanical and autonomic rhythms that shape HRV frequencies. Studies on intermediate A^uI respiratory methods have shown that speed and depth of breath affect which HRV frequency is activated. *Resonant breathing* is a standard feature in many forms of intermediate A^uI, consisting of a twelve-second respiration cycle (a deep six-second inhalation followed by a six-second exhalation). Resonant breathing tends to increase high frequency HRV, an indication of enhanced parasympathy. In contrast to resonant breathing, some forms of yogic breathing lengthen and slow respiration, stretching out the cycle to as long as a minute. This longer, slow-paced approach tends to increase low frequency HRV, generally interpreted as the sign of an attempt by autonomic central to restore parasympathetic and sympathetic balance (Peng, et al).

In addition to HRV effects, a few Mindfulness studies suggest that intermediate A^uI breathing techniques can lower inflammatory cytokines in the blood (Haenzel). The conclusions of these findings are strengthened by other large studies that connect the dots between increased HRV and low levels of inflammation in the blood. The beauty of these breathing approaches to intermediate A^uI is their simplicity. But their one-sidedness in terms of sympathetic or parasympathetic activation limits their value and impact. Resonant breathing produces a valuable effect so long as you don't need to stay alert. Its promotion of parasympathetic dominance could cause relaxation to the point of drowsiness. Conversely, the sympathetic overdrive caused by rapid breathing could induce dizziness through hyperventilation.

Side effects notwithstanding, breath-centered intermediate A^uI appears to have health benefits. As mentioned previously, these benefits can penetrate, at least temporarily, to the genomic level. Conventional exercise can accomplish similar effects in less time,

Illustration 19: Effects of Exercise Breathing, Vigorous Yoga Breathing, Resonant and Long, Slow Breathing on HRV Frequencies

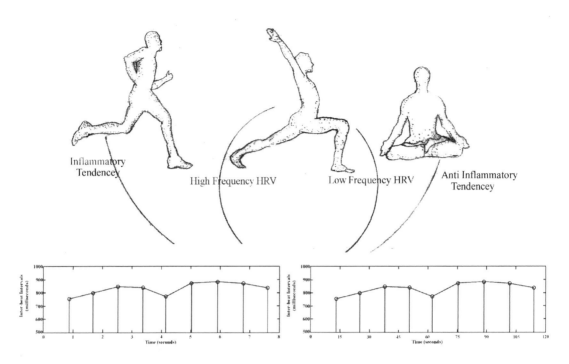

with the same limits of duration. The takeaway lesson is two-fold: 1. regularity and consistency are necessary for achieving sustainable health effects from either basic or intermediate A^uI, and 2. breathing is an essential part of all levels of A^uI.

Focus and Compassion

Unlike respiration, focus is more of an exclusive feature of intermediate A^uI. The primary way intermediate A^uI achieves focus is through guided meditation that directs attention inward to either emotions or physical processes such as respiration or heart rate. These guided meditative methods rely on concepts or images rooted in contemporary psychology, ancient traditions, or some mixture of the two. Mindfulness is probably the best known such hybridization, blending aspects of cognitive therapy with Buddhist practices that foster attention on the moment and empathy and respect for the suffering of others. Many other forms of guided meditation make use of "heart-centered" approaches grounded in other religious traditions, including Judaism, Christianity, and Aboriginal shamanism. The one trait these intermediate A^uI methods have in common is that they appeal to compassion toward the self and others. Healthcare practitioners and researchers have found this appeal to have enormous healing power. In the 20th Century, this healing phenomenon came to be known as the "Hawthorne-Placebo Effect" (HPE).

The HPE has two dimensions based on its double name. "Hawthorne" refers to a series of incidents that occurred in 1924 at an Illinois AT&T manufacturing plant called the Hawthorne Works of the Western Electric Company. After replacing burned-out lights with bulbs that were brighter, management observed that that worker productivity appeared to increase. At first the brighter lighting was assumed to have caused the uptick, but over time, management came to understand that the attention the employees received was the driving factor. From this case, and from observing its effects repeated *ad nauseum*, medicine came to recognize the healing power of human attention.

"Placebo" refers to a phenomenon that has become the gold standard for conducting medical research. To test whether or not medication has objectively measurable effects, subjects in an experiment are divided randomly into two groups. One group gets the medicine; the other gets a *placebo* (Latin for "I shall be pleasing"), usually in the form of a sugar pill. Both groups think they are getting the real deal. On average, the sugar pill turns out to improve patient outcomes by roughly thirty percent. Through these "double-blind" (nobody knows who gets what) "placebo-controlled" (the placebo-taker outcomes are compared to the medicine-taker outcomes), conventional medicine inadvertently uncovered the healing power of belief.

For a long time, conventional medical practitioners disparaged the restorative power of attention and belief. "HPE" was synonymous with snake oil and fraud. But in recent years, a growing chorus within medicine, especially among nurses, has argued that the HPE is legitimate medicine that should be woven seamlessly into a patient's experience. Top medical institutions have incorporated entire programs that teach healthcare professionals intermediate A^uI methods that openly acknowledge the helpful role of the HPE, Mindfulness being the most prominent.

These developments have helped to redeem the HPE, but the snake-oil perception remains relatively strong among many of the old guard, who feel a righteous responsibility to protect patients from false hope and exploitation. Mindfulness researchers have pushed back against this stubbornness by theorizing that the HPE is an autonomic function that has evolved out of *neuroplasticity*, the nervous system's capacity to build new interconnections. In sum, these theories hold that the human ability to self-regulate through higher executive brain functions allows for some control over the sympathetic and parasympathetic rheostats. Thus both the giver and receiver of the HPE calm, soothe, and restore themselves by dialing up the parasympathetic rheostat and dialing back the sympathetic.

The problem with this idea is that it portrays the HPE as a broad function of human nature, but it shows up only thirty percent of the time. Mindfulness advocates have attempted to answer this fair question by drilling down to the supreme level of molecular biology, and it appears that they have found a gene that may make someone susceptible to the HPE. Researchers assessed blood samples in a previous study that looked for the HPE in patients with irritable bowel syndrome (IBS). The original study distributed the IBS patients randomly among three treatment arms. In the first arm, patients were wait-listed with no treatment. The second-arm group received acupuncture therapy in a pared-down setting. The third-arm group also got acupuncture treatment but in a warm, caring environment. The genetic marker showed up most strongly in the third-arm group. Those who possessed the marker were six times more likely to respond favorably to the HPE aspects of the treatment (Hall, et al.).

The possibility of the discovery of an HPE gene has generated a great deal of excitement, since it holds the promise of helping researchers tease out the HPE from medical treatment studies. Some hypothesize that HPE gene may make someone susceptible not only to the power of belief and attention, but also to greater curiosity and open-mindedness. This could mean that the HPE gene might also be a marker of neuroplasticity, a helpful trait when trying to enhance A^uI. It may turn out that those who lack the gene are sympathetic-dominant, and are therefore inherently mistrustful and unable to relax, perpetually coiled in preparation for the proverbial lion springing out the savannah. This knowledge could help someone missing the HPE gene to manage expectations while trying to gain intermediate A^uI.

Even more interestingly, some studies suggest that HPE susceptibles can enhance HPE tendencies in those who lack the genetic marker. This kind of information might be of great benefit for large organizations with highly competitive, stressful environments. Identify and distribute the HPE susceptible population wisely and employee relations might run more smoothly.

These kinds of discoveries demonstrate the potential of intermediate $A''I$. To date, Mindfulness advocates have produced enough evidence to have convinced medical, government, and business organizations to fold Mindfulness into their educational and leadership programs. In the workplace, the Mindfulness movement has gained considerable traction as both a stress buster and management tool. Mindfulness experts regularly headline top-tier business conventions. High-tech companies like Google have their own Mindfulness faculty that provides employees with ongoing opportunities to benefit from Mindfulness methods.

Beyond the Intermediate

Within all success stories, pitfalls lurk. Resting on laurels and evolving a complacent sense of "we know what's going on" tends to discourage imagining the possibility of something greater. This complacency affects not only healthcare consumers, but also institutions that fund medical research, where novel ideas tend to be regarded as "fishing expeditions." The underlying message of this attitude is not just "we know what's going on," but rather "we may not know everything that's going on, but we know better than anyone else."

Unfortunately, this better knowledge has not included the possibility of advanced $A''I$ through the RfR, the vivid sensory impression of the pulsatile self, which gives an individual unprecedented control over health. Because the RfR is immediately sensible and novel, it fosters the belief in the power of self-healing. It also has proven superior in enhancing autonomic cardiovascular and immune oscillations in head-to-head comparison with Mindfulness. It can be summoned pretty much at will, thus making control over autonomic cardiovascular and immune oscillations a part of consciousness. At first, sitting or lying down somewhere quietly is necessary to achieve this awareness, but as experience grows, so does the freedom to trigger the RfR. It can be activated while standing or even walking. Some may even be able to sense it during vigorous exercise, though the greatest benefits derive from prolonged seated meditations.

Part 2

Advanced A^uI: Building the Pulsatile Self through RE and the RfR

Chapter 6

Advanced A^uI: Understanding and Learning to Sense the Pulsatile Self through RE

This section concentrates on teaching you RE in order to acquire advanced A^uI. As mentioned previously, there are other methods of acquiring advanced A^uI, but they take longer and involve Far Eastern concepts rooted more in religion than in science. While these features may appeal to some, RE is designed for people who want results fast that can be explained in A^uI terms. Once RE is learned and it delivers the RfR and a sense of the pulsatile self, the practitioner has a skeleton key for unlocking the superior benefits of complex exercises such as Taiji (Tai Chi). Without acquiring the RfR and a sense of the pulsatile self, however, the superior benefits of such exercise probably will remain out of reach.

RE Video Support

Chapter 6 provides text and visual instruction, including video hyperlink icons, for learning RE. An eight-session video entitled *Reflective Exercise in 8 Sessions*: *Discovering and Cultivating the Pulsatile Self* can be purchased at www.pulsatileinternational.com, where a free introduction to the video is also available.

RE and the Connection between Basic, Intermediate, and Advanced A^uI

Basic and intermediate A^uI enhance autonomic cardiovascular and immune system function through different features of evolved human biology. As discussed in Part 1, a respectable body of research has shown that both basic and intermediate A^uI can increase HRV (especially in the high frequency), reduce inflammation, and promote healthy changes in the genome that regulate the stress response.

To review, basic A^uI accomplishes these effects through our body's flight-or-fight response to muscle contraction, movement, and respiration. Applying basic A^uI by taking a twenty-to-thirty minute run, for example, triggers dominant sympathetic activity that increases heart rate, blood pressure, and elevates inflammation through wear-and-tear on the body's tissues. These heightened sympathetic effects summon a parasympathetic reaction to keep the cardiovascular system from exceeding its hydraulic and chemical limits. During rest following the run, the situation reverses itself. Sympathetic activity dials down, allowing the parasympathetic side to dominate and restore the autonomic cardiovascular and immune systems to healthy balance.

Intermediate A^uI depends on our more highly evolved social nature to restore autonomic cardiovascular and immune systems that are stuck in sympathetic overdrive. Through mental focus, feelings of goodwill toward oneself and others, and resonant breathing (roughly a twelve second respiration cycle), intermediate A^uI can evoke our latent susceptibility to the HPE, which dials down the sympathetic rheostat and dials up the parasympathetic rheostat to lower blood pressure and dampen inflammation.

We can feel the healthy effects of basic and intermediate A^uI as a general sense of wellbeing. In contrast, a person with advanced A^uI enjoys a far more specific experience that suggests the ability to sense and control the autonomic cardiovascular and immune systems in real-time, moment-to-moment. Studies conducted on RE practitioners show that significant increases in low frequency HRV and blood pressure variability (BPV) occur when the RfR is experienced. A respectable and growing body of research ties reduced levels of the chemical signatures of inflammatory reflex activation to increases in the low frequency side of the HRV spectrum (Haenzel, et al).

Despite this important difference in effect, RE builds advanced A^uI off of basic and intermediate A^uI features. RE relies on a breathing and movement to trigger sympathetic and parasympathetic responses, similar to the way low-intensity conventional exercise like slow walking with rhythmic breathing might. Like intermediate A^uI, RE also requires practitioner to concentrate not only on respiration rhythm and speed, but also on specific positions of the tongue and teeth as well as muscular tension in the jaw and lower abdominal muscular actions that are coordinated with both respiration and detailed movements. This brings awareness to autonomic cardiovascular functions and moves consciousness out of its default mode of screening out such awareness. These intermediate A^uI effects combine with those of basic A^uI to prepare the way for advanced A^uI to emerge during a meditative phase, which intensifies the autonomic nervous system's sensory capacity. This intensified sensory capacity eventually becomes the RfR, a palpable sensation that effectively allows the practitioner not only to generate robust increases in low frequency HRV, but also to channel and focus the IR on a health problem.

How RE Becomes Advanced A^uI

RE produces the advanced A^uI effect of the RfR through *classical conditioning*, the neuroplastic relationship between sensory inputs and the nervous system, first identified by the early 20th-century Russian neurologist Ivan Pavlov. In his famous experiment with a dog, Pavlov demonstrated that over time a dog's autonomic reflex to salivate at the sight and smell of food could be trained to react to a novel stimulus, like a ringing bell. Doing RE for thirty to forty-five minutes twice daily over as few as three consecutive days can condition a similar connection between the sensory dimension of the autonomic cardiovascular and immune systems (the vagus nerve in particular) and the sensory dimension of consciousness. In this way, RE evokes the RfR and builds the pulsatile self.

The Elements of RE

RE combines three elements into a single twenty to thirty minute routine. The three elements are 1. Reflective Breathing, 2. Reflective Movement, and 3. Reflective Meditation in standing, seated, and supine positions. These three elements must be learned in a step-by-step process over the span of six to eight sessions lasting thirty to forty minutes each. For best results, training sessions should happen as close together as possible, preferably within one week. With this kind of schedule, the neuroplastic changes RE promotes are less likely to be disrupted by competing behaviors that destabilize the ability to sense the pulsatile self. If you are unwilling or unable to commit to such an upfront time demand, then you should be prepared for slower and perhaps weaker effects.

Reflective Breathing

Reflective Breathing is based on an East Asian martial art technique called "reverse breathing," used to enhance power. But three highly specific, nuanced features distinguish Reflective Breathing from the general martial technique, which can vary according to teacher and/or traditional idiosyncrasies.

1. Breathing specifics (see feature 2 for visual illustration):

  - Air flows exclusively in and out through the nostrils.
  - Breathing should be "light" so that the lungs don't overfill.

- The cycle should be neither deep nor long, but rather approximately three seconds for inhalation and three seconds for exhalation.

2. Lower abdominal muscle maneuver:

- Gentle contraction in sync with the inhalation and then gentle relaxation in sync with the exhalation.

- Contractions and expansions are not forceful, but subtle, fluid, and constant.

- To the naked eye, the contractions and expansion are subtle.

Contract Lower
Abdomen on Inhalation

Relax Lower Abdomen
on Exhalation

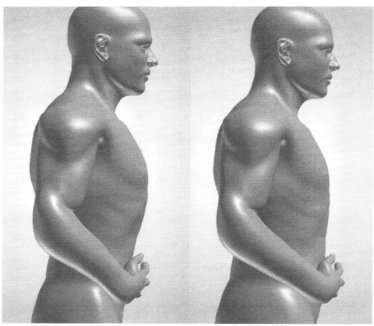

3. Tongue, teeth, and jaw position (click on hyperlink icon):

- The tongue lifts from the center into the upper palate, and the tip rests behind the front teeth.

Tongue Position

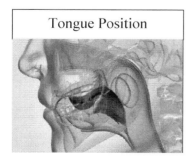

- Molars should touch lightly.
- Mastoid muscles of the jaw should flex mildly.

Reflective Movement

Once the general features of Reflective Breathing can be performed reasonably well, the next thing to learn is Reflective Movement, a four minute routine that combines Reflective Breathing with coordinated movements of the legs, arms, and hands. The entire routine is fluid and constant, but for learning purposes, it can be broken down into the following components:

1. Lower Body (waist and below)
2. Upper Body (above the waist)
3. Reflective Movements (Lower and Upper Body combined) Synced with Reflective Breathing

Lower Body: Feet, Legs, and Hips

The lower body aspects of Reflective Movement include the position of the feet and the synchronous actions of the legs and waist. The feet are spread approximately one shoulder-width, with the toes pointing straight ahead, so that the weight is distributed evenly. The routine begins with a gradual bending of the knees, coordinated with a Reflective exhalation.

Beginning Lower Body Position

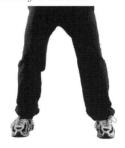

From that point until the routine is complete, the weight shifts from one leg to the other by means of forty-five degree hip rotations to the left and right in two dimensions: forward and backward. To get an understanding of how the lower body movements work, they should be practiced as an independent exercise, starting on the left side in the forward dimension.

In the forward dimension, the weight shifts in the direction of the hip rotation, so when executed to the left, the hips turn forty-five degrees left, which puts the weight primarily over the left leg. Then, with the hips maintaining the forty-five degree left angle, the weight shifts back to the right, after which the hips turn right until they are oriented in the center position.

Forward Left Lower Body

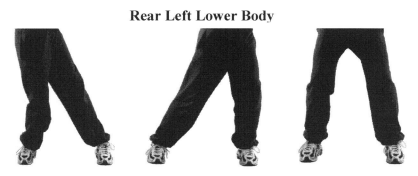

In the left-side rear dimension, the relationship between hip rotations and weight shifts reverses. When the hips rotate forty-five degrees left, the weight shifts primarily to the right. Then while maintaining the forty-five degree angle, the weight shifts back to the left, after which the hips rotate forty-five degrees right back to the central position, with the weight distributed evenly between both legs.

Rear Left Lower Body

After completing these lower body movements on the left, the process is repeated to the right side in both the forward and rear dimensions.

Forward Right Lower

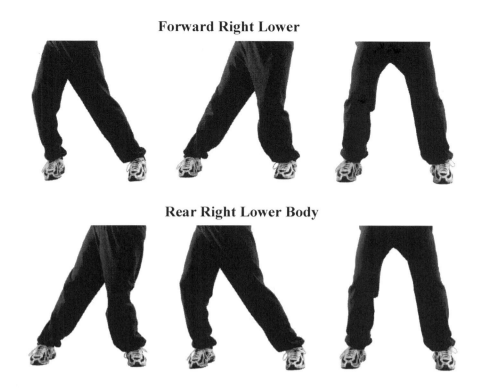

Rear Right Lower Body

Upper Body: Arms and Hand Positions and the Three Centers

The upper body aspects of Reflective Movement involve the arms and hands. Regarding the arms, all forward and lateral movement occurs through the elbow joint, which forms an angle that vacillates between 90 and 160 degrees. Hand movement happens at the wrist, either through rotating or flexing the wrist joint. The hands are open-palmed with all fingers loosely together, except for the thumbs, which should be spread apart from the rest of the hand.

Movement of Arms and Elbows, Hands and Wrists

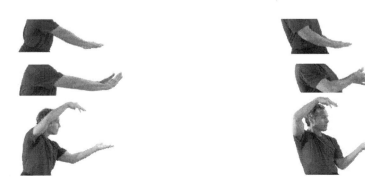

During Reflective Movement, the hands are positioned at the lower abdomen, chest, and head, defined separately as the Low, Middle, and High Centers, and collectively as the Three Centers. When held at the Low Center, the palms face downward, approximately two inches from your body. At the Middle Center, the palms face away from you, also approximately two inches from your body. At the High Center, one hand dangles a couple of inches over your head, with the palm facing downward. The other hand should be held at the center of chest, with the palm facing upward. As with the other two positions, at the high level the hands extend approximately two inches from your body.

Hand movement at the high center level is the most complex of the three, because when going from a left-side sequence of movement to the right side, the arms and hand reverse positions. A good way to keep these positions straight is to remember to tether the upward-facing hand to the direction of the movement, so that, for example, when starting a sequence to the left, the left hand will be at the chest level, with the palm facing upward. This and other positional aspects of the upper body have to be integrated smoothly with lower body movements while using Reflective Breathing.

Hand Positions of the Three Centers

Reflective Meditation

Reflective Meditation aims sensory awareness inward. Of the three RE elements, Reflective Meditation is most directly involved in the emergence of the RfR, which provides the basis for cultivating the pulsatile self. A more detailed theory of how this happens is laid out in Chapter 8

Reflective Meditation is of two kinds: Dynamic and Still. Dynamic Reflective Meditation is performed exclusively in a standing position. Still Reflective Meditation occurs while standing or while seated or reclining in a supine position on the floor.

Dynamic Reflective Meditation

Dynamic Reflective Meditation is performed in a standing position and involves either whole body or hand-and-arm movement. During these whole-body or hand-and-arm movements, the hands either remain in front of one Center or move continually from one Center to another. Dynamic Reflective Meditation produces sensations in the hands that can be traced back to internal autonomic cardiovascular and immune system *reflections*, changes in the oscillating hydraulic, electromagnetic, thermal, and acoustic forces ricocheting around in the body from the lower abdomen to the head. Repeatedly sensing these reflections with the hands is an important first step in directing the sense of touch inward to elicit the RfR and begin the development of the pulsatile self.

Middle Center   **Low Center**   **High Center**

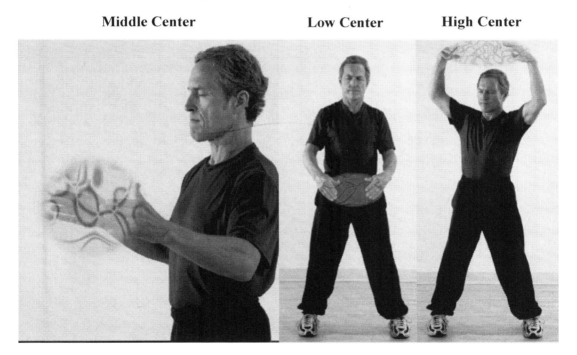

Closing Sculpt

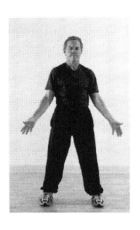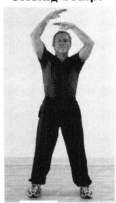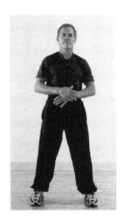

Still Reflective Meditation

Still Reflective Meditation takes two forms: Standing Reflective Meditation, which assists in the ability to sense reflections, and Seated or Supine Reflective Meditation, which essential for both sensing and working with the RfR. With mature ability to sense and manipulate the RfR, Standing Reflective Meditation becomes unnecessary, but Seated or Supine Reflective Meditation should become a fixture of the routine. It helps develop the ability to sense and move the RfR at all hours of the day, a form of behavioral prevention with enormous promise.

Standing Reflective Meditation

This still form of Reflective Meditation follows Reflective Movement and consists simply of holding the arms and the hands at the Middle Center, as though gently embracing someone. The spine is erect but not rigid, the legs straight without being taut, elbows relaxed downward toward the ribcage.

To shut out distracting stimuli, the eyes should be closed, though occasionally they can be opened to check the time throughout the two to five minutes of holding the posture. Reflective Breathing should be constant (tongue still lifted to the back of the upper gums, teeth lightly touching, jaw muscles subtly flexed).

Holding the arms in this posture affects the sensory nerves in the hands in one or two possible ways. Either the sensory nerves of the hands baste in and thus are able to feel the energetic projections of the Middle Center, or they begin to feel changes in circulation in the hands caused by holding the posture for an extended period of time. As a side benefit, the posture strengthens subtle back and core muscles that can gird and improve posture.

Standing Reflective Meditation

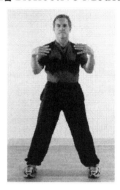

Seated or Supine Reflective Meditation

Seated or Supine Reflective Meditation is essential in experiencing the RfR. In general it is performed after Reflective Movement. As the name implies, this static phase of meditation involves either sitting in a chair or reclining on the back, face upward. In a chair, you should sit on the forward edge, away from the backrest, both feet flat on the floor. If you are tired or are uncomfortable sitting upright, try lying flat on your back. If you suffer from low-back or pelvic conditions that make such reclining uncomfortable, place a pillow under your legs.

Seated Reflective Meditation   **Reclining Reflective Meditation**

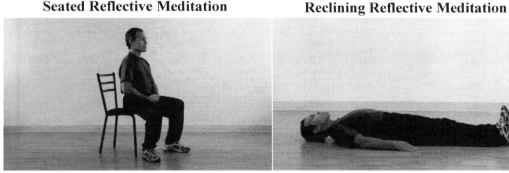

Whether seated or lying down, use Reflective Breathing. Beginning meditators should start off lightly with five-minute sessions, because sitting still and concentrating on Reflective Breathing takes practice. If drowsiness sets in, just take a nap and wake up spontaneously. Afterwards, you should feel more refreshed.

For more experienced meditators, and as a novice's ability to concentrate and sit comfortably increases, the sessions should last a full twenty minutes. This is as essential to getting and working effectively with the RfR. The RfR may emerge abruptly during Seated or Reclining Meditation, as it did in my case, with a vascular sensation that shoots straight from the lower abdomen into the head. Or it may begin subtly with a rising and falling sensation that follows your inhalations and exhalations. As the sensation comes to feel more vascular, the sinuses may clear. Either exhilaration or deep relaxation may follow. In either case, the sensation is new, and the research conducted thus far, the thousand-plus anecdotal cases, and centuries of experience accumulated by the "wisdom traditions" of inwardly-directed Far Eastern cultures suggest that the phenomenon marks enhanced control over the mechanisms the body uses to generate health.

Start blazing your own pathway to sustainable health with the RE instructional video *Reflective Exercise in 8 Sessions*: *Discovering and Cultivating the Pulsatile Self*. This helpful video can be purchased for streaming at www.pulsatileinternational.com.

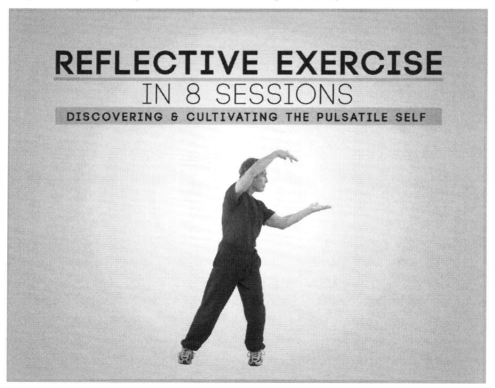

Chapter 7
The Theory of Advanced A^uI, the RfR, and the Pulsatile Self

RE moves the needle from intermediate to advanced A^uI by developing in the RE practitioner the RfR: the ability to sense, channel, and focus the IR as a cardiovascular sensation, which can be measured as an increase in low frequency HRV. This ability emerges from repeating the combined RE behaviors of Reflective Breathing, Movement, and Meditation, which connects consciousness, the sense of touch, and the sensory dimension of the autonomic cardiovascular and immune systems.

Dynamic Reflective Meditation directly activates the sense of touch through the hands. The sensations that the hands pick up can be attributed to at least two kinds of cardiovascular reflections regulated by the autonomic rheostats. One possibility is that the sensations may be a tactile impression of the body's thermo-electromagnetic reflections that project approximately six inches into the airspace surrounding the brain, heart, and lower abdominal viscera. Sensing these energies would activate the brain's hand-sensory nerve center located in the parietal lobe. This possibility seems more like reality once the RfR emerges. When that happens, not only can the hands feel energetic projections from the head, chest, and lower abdomen, but also using the hands to engage those energetic projections can effect internal sensations such as pressure changes in the sinuses, pain relief and motility in the visceral organs, and the intensity of oscillations of the autonomic cardiovascular and immune systems.

The other possibility is that hand sensation is more of a shadow effect created by the hydraulics of the autonomic cardiovascular system, especially in the early stages of RE training, when the practice of Reflecting the Middle Center begins. Holding the arms at chest level for several minutes has an unquestionable basic A^uI effect on peripheral blood pressure. From this perspective, the practitioner could be sensing fluctuations in the diameter of the blood vessels in the hands that are responding to the basic A^uI behaviors of using back, shoulder, and arm muscles to hold the arms in an elevated position for several minutes and then moving the hands to detect what feels like thermo-electromagnetic energy. When the practitioner goes from holding the arms still to moving them, the muscle groups in the arms, shoulders, and back can cycle between relaxation and tension, changing the internal blood pressure dynamic within the vasculature of the hands and arms. Tactile neurons of the hands and sympathetic nerve fibers within the smooth muscle lining the arteries provide the means of sensing within the hands' blood vessels these pressure shifts, which the barometric sensory receptors in the aortic arch and carotid artery detect and communicate directly to autonomic central.

Illustration 20: Two Possible Sources of Hand Sensations during Reflective Meditation

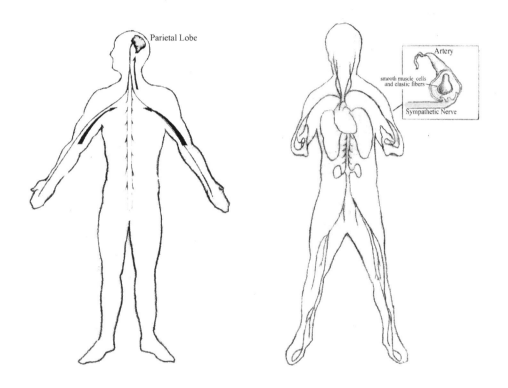

These two sensations may occur separately or simultaneously. In either case, feeling in the hands will activate the brain's hand-sensory region in the parietal lobe. During Dynamic Reflective Meditation, this nerve center remains active and mingles with the basic and intermediate $A^u I$ effects wrought by Reflective Breathing and Movement. Like Pavlov continually ringing the bell before serving mouthwatering food to his dog subject, the RE practitioner constantly activates the sense of touch while subjecting the autonomic cardiovascular system to the influence of basic and intermediate $A^u I$ effects. In this way, RE practice begins to merge the two nerve pathways and transform autonomic nervous system into a sensory organ that can detect and eventually influence internal hydraulic shifts.

Illustration 21: How RE Transforms the Autonomic Cardiovascular System into a Sensory Organ

RE routine

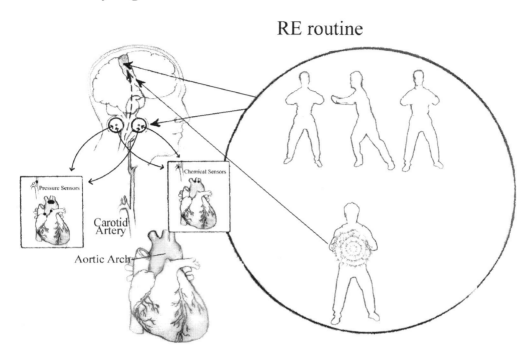

The RfR and the Sensory Vagus

The aspect of the autonomic nervous system most likely influenced by Reflective Breathing during Reflective Meditation is the vagus nerve, the major arm of the parasympathetic rheostat with important sensory ties to the sympathetic rheostat. This sympathetic sensory connection could be the basis for feeling the RfR, and two subtle features of Reflective Breathing provide the means: the slight muscular tension in the tongue and jaw and the constant cycle of contraction of lower abdominal muscles synced with the in-breath and relaxation of those muscles synced with the out-breath. The pharyngeal branch of the vagus nerve projects into both the jaw muscle and tongue, and so the slight tension in the jaw and tongue likely stimulates sensory feedback from those vagal projections, as well as from the laryngeal branch of the vagus nerve that extends below into the throat and thyroid gland. The tongue's sensory capacity could combine with pharyngeal vagal activation to contribute to the ability to feel the RfR in the mouth and head.

Illustration 22: The Pharyngeal-Laryngeal Effects of Reflective Breathing

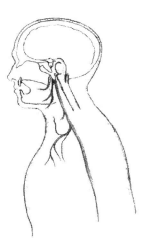

The lower abdominal muscular maneuver of Reflective Breathing likely applies stimulating pressure on the immense cluster of abdominal vagal nerve fibers that, in turn, are surrounded by a vast nerve cloud known as the enteric nervous system (ENS).

These two nerve constellations constitute an "abdominal brain," constantly communicating with each other and the upper brain, including the sensory aspect of nervous system (the "peripheral nervous system"). Stomach and intestinal pain, nausea, butterflies, and other commonly felt gut-centered sensations attest to the abdominal brain's sensory capacity, known in medicalese as *interoception*. These interoceptive visceral sensations register not only through the sensory aspect of the nervous system, but also though the vagus nerve's sympathetic arm, which also governs the actions of the IR's lymphocyte army, concentrated in the gastrointestinal tract. Combined with jaw and tongue activation of the pharyngeal vagal branch, the lower abdominal muscular maneuver may heighten the abdominal brain's sympathetic sensory capacity so that it

Illustration 23: The ENS and the Effects of Reflective Breathing on the Abdominal Vagus Nerve Plexus

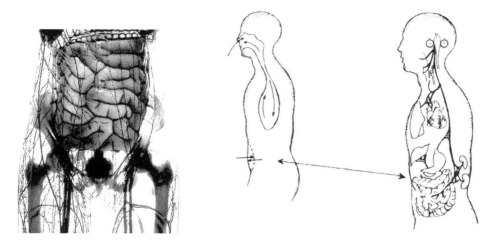

begins to detect and to shape autonomic cardiovascular and immune system activity.

Sensing Aortic Reflections

The RfR typically emerges during Reflective Meditation as a vascular sensation that runs from lower abdomen to head along a vertical pathway that coincides with the central arterial tree. This cardiovascular pathway has two major autonomic feeds: sympathetic nerves, which line the smooth muscle of the central artery (as well as that of lesser arteries), and the vagus nerve, which attaches to the arterial tree, as well as all the major organs in the trunk. Through Reflective Breathing combined with the other elements of RE, the RE practitioner likely foments the RfR by recruiting and honing the sensory potential of these two autonomic cardiovascular inputs.

Of the two autonomic feeds to the central artery, the vagal attachments probably are more directly responsible for the emergence of the RfR. Numerous studies have shown that the vagus nerve communicates heartbeat behavior not only to autonomic central, but also to higher executive brain centers. The upshot of these studies is that vagal communication of heartbeat behavior, or *heart evoked potential* (HEP), can be modulated by learning resonant breathing patterns that increase both low and high frequency HRV. The principal vagal centers that deliver these HEP's are the barometric and chemical sensory receptors in the aortic arch and carotid artery (Chiesa, et al). The RfR likely uses the same vagal mechanisms, but with enhanced sensory capacity that allows detection of a greater array of forces produced by the cardiovascular system.

One of those forces may be the constant noisy propulsion of blood payloads, up and down the arterial column, the structure of which varies in three key places: the upper chest (including the neck and shoulder), the middle abdomen, and the pelvis. Whenever a blood payload strikes one of these variable structures, "reflections," or echo-like aftershocks, occur and propagate throughout the body's vasculature. With their sensory potential enhanced through RE, the aortic and carotid vagal barometric and chemical sensory receptors could become the equivalent of internal fingers, capable of feeling reflections at the upper reflection site. As the RE practitioner's sense of the RfR deepens, the aortic and carotid sensors also may combine with the sympathetic nerves in the arterial

Illustration 24: Three Reflection Sites and their Proximity to Aortic Sensors and Sympathetic Arterial Nerves

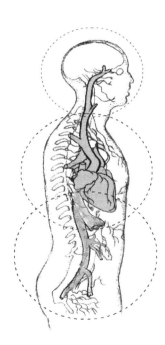

wall to provide the capacity to feel and begin to manipulate oscillations in the diameter of the central artery. With this deeper sense of the RfR, the RE practitioner is able to massage the pulsatile self into being.

Another likely source of the RfR's internal tactile intensification is the hand-sensory nerve center, activated during Dynamic Reflective Meditation. The combined RE elements could condition a neuroplastic connection between the hand-sensory nerve center and the sensory aspect of the vagus nerve, effectively interfusing tactile and autonomic neuro-biology. The validity of this explanation strengthens as a sense of the RfR deepens, and the practitioner can intensify internal sensation of the pulsatile self during Dynamic Reflective Meditation by passing the hands through the air along the arterial pathway of the body from head to lower abdomen. Of the Three Centers, the high one is the most susceptible to hand engagement and manipulation. In fact, by aiming the palms or the index and middle fingers at the temples and then circling them repeatedly, a practitioner can change the sense of pressure inside the sinuses. The hands and fingers can be used in this way to open the sinuses if they are congested.

Illustration 25: Interfusion of the Hand-sensory Nerve Center and the Sensory Vagus and Using the Hands to Affect Pressure in the Head

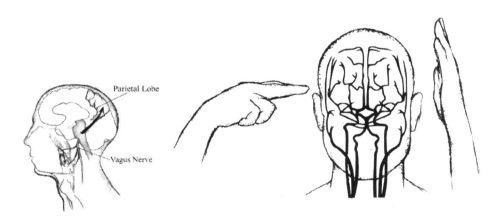

These claims are not mere theoretical speculations. Cardiovascular devices with low-pressure sensors can detect arterial reflections and use them to determine HRV and BPV. In fact, the two University of Virginia HRV studies on RE relied on such a device. Both experiments support the hypothesis that the RfR constitutes the ability to produce increases in HRV that consensus research has shown mark resilient health and enhanced immune function. One study used the device to compare the HRV measurements of fourteen RE practitioners during Seated Reflective Meditation with those of eighteen Mindfulness and Transcendental Meditation practitioners. The RE group experienced significant increases in low frequency HRV and BPV, while the Mindfulness and Transcendental group showed no significant HRV or BPV shifts (Rich, et al. "Assessment of Cardiovascular Parameters before and after Meditation").

Illustration 26: Sample Measurement of HRV and BPV Increases during RfR (starting approximately at 200)

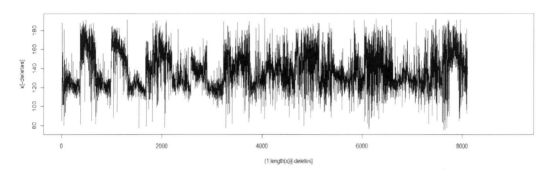

The second study used the same device to study the emergence of the RfR in a group of University of Virginia varsity swimmers who learned RE over a period of eight days and then were tested for HRV shifts once a month for three months. Swimmers who reported feeling the RfR also recorded significant increases in low frequency HRV compared to those who reported a lack or absence of RfR sensation (Rich, et al. "Assessment of Cardiovascular Parameters during Meditation with Mental Targeting in Swimmers").

Separate research has shown repeatedly that increased low frequency HRV indicates modulation of both the IR and the aortic barometric and chemical receptors.

The two studies tie the RfR to important health-creating features of the autonomic cardiovascular and immune systems, but the differences in results merit comment. The experiment that examined novice RE practitioners found only an increase in low frequency HRV as their sense of the RfR emerged during training. The study that compared the cardiovascular dynamics of more seasoned RE practitioners to Mindfulness veterans showed that the RE practitioners experienced significant increases not only in low frequency HRV, but also in BPV, an effect that can be explained by the basic A^uI effects of respiration. Measurements of continuous blood pressure have shown BPV decreases on the in-breath and increases on the out-breath. But the comparative study also found that the seasoned RE practitioners experienced an increase in the low-to-high frequency HRV ratio, something previous research on the HRV effects of meditation has not shown. This increased ratio means that the upsurge in low frequency HRV was significantly larger than that of high frequency HRV, generally considered to be driven by respiration. This greater low-to-high frequency HRV ratio suggests that the increased low frequency BPV during meditation may have been caused not by basic A^uI respiratory effects, but by the deeper autonomic process of restoring cardiovascular pressure to equilibrium, described in Chapter 3. Based on the cumulative evidence, sensory control of the aortic barometric and chemical receptors makes for a plausible explanation. Because research on other forms of meditation has not shown this HRV effect, it is reasonable to use this ratio of low-to-high frequency HRV as a unique marker of a mature sense of the RfR.

To assist the RE trainee in verifying the subjective but powerful sense of the RfR, *Pulsatile International* (www.pulsatileinternational.com) provides for download the "RfR-app," a software program that looks for the signature HRV effects of the RfR. With instructions provided on the app as well as from this book and the RE video (also available for download from www.pulsatileinternational.com), the RfR-app can help you to visually corroborate your sense of the RfR emerging from your RE training. Using the RfR-app in this way helps objectively affirm that you are not only generating health benefits by increasing both low frequency HRV, but also establishing deeper autonomic cardiovascular and immune system control, once you are able to manifest an increase in both low frequency BPV and low-to-high frequency HRV ratio. These latter two signals indicate a strong state of pulsatile being.

The RfR and IR

The IR's center is located in the vast cluster of gastrointestinal lymph glands, which the vagal dendrites project directly into. Through these projections AutCentCom receives messages from and issues orders to the lymphocyte army holed up inside the glands.

Illustration 27: Vagal Dendrites Penetrating Lymph Gland

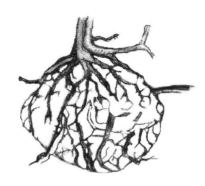

On the basic and intermediate A^uI levels, cardiovascular stimulation can trigger immune effects—the way, for example, exercise dials up the sympathetic rheostat and increases levels of pro-inflammatory flame-throwers. Advanced A^uI works the same connection, but rooted more deeply in an awareness of the immediate, pulsatile nature of the autonomic cardiovascular and immune systems, made possible by an enhanced sensory capacity of the vagus nerve. That awareness is the RfR, which through vagal activation affects both cardiovascular oscillations and the abdominal brain (gut-centered vagal nerves and the ENS). By absorbing the chemical messages from heightened abdominal brain activity, lymphocyte soldiers garrisoned in gastrointestinal glands become turbocharged. Molecular studies show that such vagal and ENS chemical messages energize lymphocytes and impart to them the potential to pass those signals to other cells, which they seek out by migrating out of their glandular barracks in the gastrointestinal tract and into other areas of the body (Pert).

This migration is made possible by a large vein leading from the gastrointestinal tract, to the spleen and liver, to the heart, to the lungs, then to the heart again, which feeds directly into the aortic and carotid arteries. The vagus nerve attaches all along this blood pathway. Of particular note is the vagal contact with the lungs and the spleen. Both organs play important roles in autonomic immune system function, but the spleen's immune function is especially noteworthy. It manufactures a specific class of lymphocyte soldier that scouts for problems. If enhanced vagal activity can mobilize the lymphocyte army in the gastrointestinal tract, then it likely can do the same with lymphocyte scouts through the vagal contact point with the spleen.

Illustration 28: The Venous Pathway and Mobilization of Lymphocytes through Heightened Sensory Activation of the Vagus Nerve and the ENS

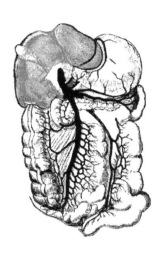
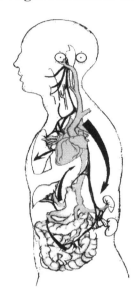

In addition to mobilizing the lymphocyte army, RfR-intensified sensory vagal capacity at attachments along the venous pathway could enable the detection and even control of blood moving up from the lower abdomen to the spleen and liver. Control over blood flow could happen through the RfR's influence on heart rate and central arterial diameter, which necessarily affects the volume and speed of blood flow through the gastrointestinal vein. Through manipulation of the autonomic rheostats, the RfR could speed the heart and dilate the aortic arch, which would increase the volume and speed of blood throughout the veins, a change in cardiovascular hydraulics that the abdominal brain might be able to detect.

Once the sense of the RfR becomes strong, the RE practitioner can use it to monitor and affect these hydraulic changes in the cardiovascular system through basic $A^{u}I$

modifications of Reflective Breathing. As discussed earlier in Part 1, the mechanics of respiration oscillate heart rate and central pressure. The RE practitioner can use those same mechanics to heighten feeling of hydraulic changes caused by the RfR. Lengthening the in-breaths of the respiration cycle creates a sense of fullness in the head. In contrast, a lengthened out-breath decreases head fullness and allows a sense of falling pressure down the vertical pathway to the lower abdomen. In this way, the RE practitioner deepens a sense of the pulsatile self.

This anatomical, neuro-biological explanation accounts for how my initial pulsatile leap turned a respiratory infection into an *exfection*. Heightened sensory vagus nerve secretions mustered lymphocytes in the gastrointestinal tract and spleen out into the venous pathway leading to the lungs and heart. From the heart, the newly charged soldiers jettisoned into the central artery and up into the carotid artery, which encircles and feeds into the sinus cavity. Once in the sinuses, they went into action, tagging the infectious agent, corroding its many replicates, and dragging their bits into narrow lymphatic channels wending through increasingly superficial layers of tissue. Along the way, germ-bearing lymphocytes triggered sympathetic fibers and sensory nerves, making surrounding muscles flutter and spasm. Finally, what was left of the germ warfare ended up on the skin as hives or pimples.

My first pulsatile leap was not unique. In the latter 1980's, many Chinese who were practicing similar exercises reported to me the same capacity to eliminate respiratory infection symptoms. Since then, not only have I repeatedly self-treated respiratory infections, but also hundreds of other RE practitioners have done the same. Some of them have agreed graciously to provide video testimonials that are available for viewing at www.pulsatileinternational.com.

Testimonials are nice, but faith healers and practitioners of many other spiritual traditions also use personal testimonies to make claims that far exceed those made here. This is one reason why research on RE is important. The first RE study examined whether or not practicing RE would have an effect on the rate of upper respiratory infection (URI) in members of the University of Virginia varsity swim team. The training endured by competitive swimmers creates such extraordinarily high levels of physical and psychological stress that their immune systems become suppressed, thus making them susceptible to URI's, a tendency shared by other high-intensity athletes and elite soldiers. The study found seventy percent fewer reported URI's in swimmers who practiced more frequently compared to those who practiced less frequently during the height of the competitive season, when swimmers tend to succumb to sickness (Wright, et al). The previously described HRV study matched a significant increase in low frequency HRV with a sense of the RfR in swimmers. Because low frequency HRV indicates activation of the IR, this second study provides a reason why RE practice protected swimmers against URI.

Another research project bolstered these findings. A U.S. Army nurse earning her PhD at the University of Virginia decided to do her dissertation on the effects of RE training on military veterans suffering from mild traumatic brain injury (m-TBI). In the case of TBI, "mild" signifies only that the sufferer isn't bed-ridden. Debilitating headaches, neuropathy, anxiety, insomnia, and post-traumatic stress disorder (PTSD) are the main m-TBI symptoms, which stem both directly and indirectly from dysfunction of the IR, the autonomic cardiovascular system, and a host of undetermined factors. The nurse recruited six veterans with m-TBI who agreed to undergo RE training while temporarily residing in rehabilitation facility that specialized in treating TBI. One recruit was dropped because of non-compliance, but the five who completed the RE training got benefits that exceeded expectations. All five got the RfR, and four used it to control their symptoms, including headache, neuropathy, anxiety, and insomnia. The nurse conducted exit interviews with the participants and included excerpts in the study, which was published in 2013. One veteran reported that "'the pulse had gotten to my head where I actually hit [it] and had the brain injury. . . .I've had it come up and it felt like, it felt like a big knot of pressure and then once I [brought] that pulse up to my head it felt like it just all evenly flowed away and then I didn't have [any] pain in my head.'" Another veteran described a similar reaction when he was experiencing a migraine headache. "'I had a real bad migraine when we started. I told him [Alton] about it and then, about halfway through the meditation of bringing that pulse up into my head and down, I felt the relief of pressure and ever since then my headaches [have] been gone.'" One study participant who had gained the ability to control his headaches and discontinue his pain medication said that when he was first told about RE, he thought to himself "'that's bull crap.' But now that I've gotten this deep into it, for me to be able to take away a headache on my own by just controlling blood flow going to my brain … that tells me right there I don't need an Excedrin or a Tylenol or some kind of drug to get rid of that'" (Yost, et al).

The veterans' descriptions of pressure changes in head suggest that some of the benefit the veterans gained were the result of the RfR's autonomic cardiovascular dimension, which will be discussed in a later chapter as an aspect of a deeper level of RE. But inflammation also plays a major role in producing TBI symptoms, so the RE/m-TBI study strengthens the observations of the relationship between the RfR and IR in the experiment with swimmers.

Two recent medical discoveries offer a window into how the RfR might restore balance to the IR in such apparently disparate conditions as m-TBI and URI. Both discoveries revealed heretofore unknown micro-lymphatic channels that connect the brain's cerebrospinal fluid (CSF) and the immune system. These findings are at odds with orthodox neuroscience, which has always held that the so-called "blood-brain barrier" prevented the kind of immune system interplay that now appears to be the case. Tiny lymphatic vessels in the dural sinus cavity and the nose that drain CSF and blood from the

Illustration 29: Micro-Lymphatics and Blood Vessels of Dural Sinus and Nose

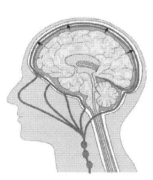

brain to the jugular vein also carry lymphocytes (Louveau, et al; Liu, et al). These passageways provide the physical means for the immune system to interact with both the cerebrospinal fluid and brain tissue.

It is entirely feasible that having learned to sense the pulsatile self, especially in the region of the sinus cavity, the veterans were using inadvertently this autonomic cardiovascular-immune nexus to dampen the chronic inflammation driving at least some of their m-TBI symptoms. When I clobbered my URI the first time I experienced the RfR, I had to have been activating the same lymphatic tubules to clear my nasal passages and sinuses. Varsity swimmers who reduced their URI symptoms most likely were doing the same thing.

Taken together, investigations into the effects of RE practice and the RfR underline the connection between imbalances in cardiovascular dynamics and in the IR, supporting the theory presented in this chapter. But they also shine a light into the two most impressive outcomes I have ever seen RE practice produce.

Chapter 8

Big Outcomes, Big Implications

At age thirty-six, a former Marine was diagnosed with a ninety-eight percent blocked carotid artery. Doctors opened the blockage with angioplasty and then for several years treated him with cholesterol-busting drugs that ultimately proved ineffective. Once an active man who was a competitive cyclist and a practicing black belt in Tae Kwan Do, he had been reduced to a shadow of his once powerful self. His doctors concluded that he had inherited coronary artery disease from his father and that the only thing they could offer was continued drug treatment until surgery became necessary.

Six years later, out of desperation, he turned to RE, and after a month of diligent practice, he experienced his pulsatile leap. While reclining one afternoon in his easy chair, the RfR came to life and traveled up the vascular pathway into his upper chest and neck. His chest seemed to expand from within, and a warm fullness traveled up into his face. His eyes inexplicably welled with tears.

The next day he worked for two hours in his yard, which he previously could do for only ten minutes before having to rest. Then he took down his old racing bicycle and rode for several miles, a feat he had not been able to perform for over six years. When he had his cholesterol markers checked out by his doctor, he and the doctor were astounded to see that all the formerly sky-high indicators had returned to acceptably healthy levels. To this day, this man remains vital and is able to benefit from directing the RfR along more advanced pathways to be discussed in the next chapter.

Another impressive outcome I witnessed involved a thirty-eight year-old woman with stage-four, metastatic breast cancer. Her sense of desperation was greater than that of the former Marine. In the vast majority of cases, stage-four cancer results in death within a year's time, because at stage four the cancer has spread throughout the body. In her case, cancer originating in the breast had migrated to her lungs and hip bone. After maximum doses of chemotherapy and radiation failed to eliminate the cancer, her doctors concluded that the best she could hope for was to survive another eighteen months.

Within the third week of RE training, she began to use reflections in her hands to feel inside her body. She claimed she could provoke turbulence near a tumor site in her lungs, which resulted in a subtle "popping" sensation. Two weeks later, when she returned to her doctor for examination, x-rays showed that the lung tumor appeared to be dead, a mass of scar tissue. Though encouraged, the doctor noted that tumor on the hip bone was still active and suggested that whatever had caused the lung tumor to die was more fluke than cure. But after four additional months of consistent RE practice, the hip-bone tumor also turned to scar tissue.

She remained tumor-free for six more years, far more time than her original eighteen-month prognosis had given her, but eventually the cancer returned and took her life. When she got the news that the cancer had returned, she reconnected with me to see what could be done. The conversation revealed that she repeatedly had yo-yoed in her RE practice since getting her original good news. She would stop practicing altogether, but whenever her regular visits to her doctor revealed an elevation in her cancer markers, she resumed RE practice until the markers dropped, after which she would discontinue practice again.

These two cases illustrate two important factors regarding disease, the RfR, and the pulsatile self. The first seems rather obvious. To combat any disease, but especially a chronic, lethal one, cultivation of the pulsatile self through consist experience of the RfR must pervade the life of the person suffering from the disease. While certainly no guarantee of conquering something as daunting as cancer or coronary artery disease, integration of the pulsatile self into daily life through constant activation of the RfR optimizes the chances to survive longer and in better health. This sometimes may seem impossible. Consider how difficult it is for many to shoehorn basic $A''I$ into their lives. Nonetheless, to reap the full benefits of advanced $A''I$, sacrifices in terms of time and energy have to be made. To assist those who have this problem, strategies for integrating all levels of $A''I$ are taken up in the next chapter.

The second factor these two cases illustrate is that experiencing consistently the pulsatile self through the RfR upended disease processes that strong evidence has shown are caused by inflammatory imbalances. The changes that occurred in inflammatory markers in the blood when each person diligently practiced support this claim. This raises another important question: what caused the inflammatory imbalance?

The Link between Infection and Serious Disease

Over the past two decades, mounting evidence has linked infectious microbes to heart disease, some cancers, diabetes, and other chronic, mortal health problems. Regarding coronary artery disease, Chlamydia pneumonia (C. pneumonia), a common respiratory bacterium, has come under increasing suspicion. C. pneumonia is an intracellular microbe. It penetrates a human cell (a specific type of lymphocyte), takes over its metabolic process, and forces the cell to produce cholesterol as a food source for the bacterium. Evidence that the germ directly causes coronary artery disease has been spotty. Some studies have shown a link while others have not. Even so, coronary artery disease has been reclassified from essentially a plumbing problem to an inflammatory one, strengthening the possibility of infectious causation.

As for cancer, strong evidence connects infection to some varieties. Helicobacter pylori and hepatitis C can cause gastrointestinal and liver cancers, and the human papilloma virus has been declared responsible for all cervical cancer and some oral and esophageal cancers.

There is no way to determine whether or not infectious microbes were behind the cases of atherosclerosis and metastatic breast cancer that the RfR helped to resolve. But if that were the case, then the explanation for how the RfR routed both diseases would be the same as that for how my initial pulsatile leap transformed a respiratory infection into an *exfection*. In fact, in both instances, each person reported feeling symptoms directly and indirectly related to the resolution of his and her disease. The man suffering from atherosclerosis described a sense of his central artery "opening," as though a cohort of flame- and fire-hoser lymphocytes had flushed out and eliminated the offender, hiding in the cellular walls of the upper aorta. The removal of the clot-forming pest left the vessel freer to transport energy-rich blood to the head and the rest of the body, restoring his sense of vitality.

The woman with metastatic breast cancer said she was able to sense one of her tumors "pop," as though a contingent of well-armed lymphocytes had identified and burst the cancerous mass. She also repeatedly reported feeling pain in a large tumor on her hip bone, suggesting that both pro-inflammation, which cancer typically weakens, and activation of sympathetic dimension of the vagus nerve were at work destroying tumor cells that x-rays eventually would show to be scar tissue.

That infection was the sole driver of these two diseases is a tempting conclusion, but other factors were surely at work. Stress was a big one. Both people confided that they were under a great deal of stress prior to the diagnosis of their health problems. After they got their diagnosis, the situation just got worse, which strengthened their diseases. Their situation underlines the complex reciprocal relationship between stress and health problems that may have an infectious microbial component. Understanding this relationship is crucial to A^uI.

Stress and Microbes: the Left and Right Hands of Inflammatory Imbalance

Like *adrenaline* and *cardiovascular*, the term *stress* has crossed over from medicine into commonplace speech, largely because medicine has identified it as a widespread health threat. The reason stress poses such a problem stems from the million or so years of natural selection that favored the survival of those with dialed-up sympathetic rheostats, which enabled swift responses to physical danger and thus the chance to live and reproduce another day. A contemporary environment, at least in a developed country, neutralizes almost all physical threats, leaving only relatively vague, remote problems to worry about: work deadlines, overdue bills, social discomforts, and so on. In the absence of life-threatening foes, these lesser, more abstract concerns become the default stand-ins for the actual threats our sympathetically inclined autonomic nervous systems have evolved in response to. This mismatch between evolution and perceived threat can imbalance the cardiovascular and immune systems. Left unchecked, these imbalances raise the risk of developing serious diseases, such as hypertension, stroke, cancer, and diabetes.

How this sympathetic imbalance promotes these diseases has not been sorted out entirely, but with A^uI a credible understanding can be pieced together. Since the sympathetic rheostat promotes speed, constriction, and heat in the cardiovascular and immune systems, a sympathetically inclined autonomic nervous system likely leads to increased cellular breakdown through wear and tear. This eventually could cause blood vessels to atrophy (hypertension) or rupture (stroke). Cellular disintegration would summon higher numbers of flame-thrower lymphocytes, causing AutCentCom to call up fire-hoser lymphocytes and anti-inflammatory hormones to restore balance. Under the flight-or-fight circumstances in which the autonomic immune system evolved, this oscillation would resolve quickly once the physical danger passed. But with unresolved chronic stress, sympathetic preponderance eventually flattens the IR's capacity to oscillate. In an effort to correct the sympathetic imbalance, levels of the anti-inflammatory hormone cortisol remain high and at some undetermined tipping point suppress the pro-inflammatory immune response. Lingering high concentrations of cortisol can intensify cellular disintegration, creating a mess for the IR's suppressed pro-inflammatory response to clean up.

These autoimmune-disruptive effects of chronic stress enhance susceptibility to infection and possibly the development of cancer. Microbes that have evolved defenses against the lymphocyte army or early-stage cancers can invade and destabilize the IR indefinitely, producing autoimmune symptoms such as allergies, as well as fatigue, insomnia, and depression, all of which can increase stress and further degrade the cardiovascular and immune systems.

Both basic and intermediate $A''I$ can help to counter some of the internal conditions driving chronic stress, though through different channels. Basic $A''I$ such as conventional exercise approximates flight-fight conditions, providing an outlet for sympathetic expression and a post-workout parasympathetic counter-expression. On the other hand, intermediate $A''I$ methods such as Mindfulness redresses stress-induced autonomic imbalance by turning up the parasympathetic rheostat through resonant breathing, attention on the moment, and compassionate focus. As mentioned earlier, both exercise and Mindfulness have been shown to reduce both cardiovascular and genomic markers of stress within two months of committed practice.

Though basic and intermediate $A''I$ are useful tools in combating the effects of chronic stress, they are not panaceas. Neither works directly on the IR. For that, advanced $A''I$ is needed. Advanced $A''I$ enhances the IR's capacity to oscillate, as demonstrated when my initial pulsatile leap ate the germ that had given me a terrible head cold and then regurgitated it as patch of hives. Those effects of the RfR on infection, combined with the HRV studies, suggest that advanced $A''I$ triggers a large IR oscillation that begins with a strong pro-inflammatory response, most likely the result of heightened interoception of the abdominal brain and its ties into the IR through the sympathetic dimension of the vagus nerve. In turn, this strong sympathetic, pro-inflammatory start naturally triggers a parasympathetic, anti-inflammatory response. Sensing the RfR conceivably could speed the cycle of flame-thrower (pro-inflammatory) and fire-hoser (anti-inflammatory) response to infection and restore balance to the autonomic cardiovascular and immune systems. In this way those who put in the time to cultivate the pulsatile self can shorten the duration of and even eliminate disease symptoms.

Pacifying Germs through the Pulsatile Self

Enhanced interoception in the abdomen brought about by experiencing the pulsatile self could lead to increased control over the IR's acute response to infectious microbes floating in the air or lying in wait. But what about the huge number of microorganisms that are already inside, located mostly in the lining of the gastrointestinal tract? This vast indigenous germ mass is known as the *microbiome*, and it shows a biological complexity and integrity not only within itself, but also with our bodies. These germs, many of which have not yet been classified, appear to work together to help out in basic matters such as breaking down and metabolizing food for energy, a process they carry out by receiving and transmitting the same molecular signals used by the IR and autonomic cardiovascular system. Because of its size (estimated to weigh between three and four pounds!) and apparent complementary function within the body, this colony of benign germs has been called a neglected "organ."

To make up for this neglect, in 2008 the National Institute of Health launched "The Human Microbiome Project" (HMP) to begin classifying and defining microorganisms associated with human health and disease. Essentially an extension of the methods used in the Human Genome Project, the HMP plans to sequence the genomes of as many human microbiomic germs as they can find and to put that information into a giant database. So far the HMP has identified germs that promote obesity by using molecular signals to manipulate the abdominal brain's connection to autonomic functions such as appetite. These germs can affect not only how much, but also what a person eats. One kind thrives when its host consumes a diet rich in red meat, and in turn secretes a substance that triggers a pro-inflammatory response from the IR. Elevated levels of pro-inflammation could induce sickness symptoms, including anxiety, insomnia, and depression, all problems that can lead to overeating and eventually to obesity, roundly considered a health threat linked to heart disease, cancer, and diabetes.

Microorganisms that permanently infest the body also can affect other areas of human behavior that can undermine health. One such troublemaking germ is *Toxoplasma gondii* (Toxo for short), a mouse-borne protozoan that is widespread in humans primarily through exposure to cat feces. Toxo has been linked to relatively mild cognitive problems such as attention deficit disorder, as well as to serious mental conditions such as bi-polar disorder and schizophrenia. Weaker evidence (but fascinating nonetheless) indicates that Toxo might be capable of manipulating complex sexual behavior in order to propagate itself. One study found that the scent of cat urine aroused people infected with Toxo. A similar study correlated characteristics associated both directly and indirectly with promiscuity and Toxo infection (McCauliff).

As it unfurls further, the HMP's efforts to tell the microbiomic story is likely to reveal more bad actors involved in health problems. Solutions appear to be headed in two directions. One direction is based on natural probiotics, which encourages the growth of good microbiomic actors that can outcompete the bad. For example, studies have shown that when red meat is restricted and replaced with foods rich in vegetable fiber, the numbers of the pro-inflammatory-generating microbes drop, while the numbers of germs that promote anti-inflammation increase. Another probiotic approach introduces good-guy germs directly into the gastrointestinal tract via stool transplant, a process accomplished by harvesting good germs from the bowel movements of healthy individuals that are then refined and put into a capsule that can be swallowed.

The other direction follows the path of bioengineering and is most likely favored by the HMP: a quest for drugs and genetically engineered microbes to correct microbiomic health problems. This approach makes a great deal of sense on an immediate level, but it may become problematic in view of the way external solutions generally tend to generate both costs and new problems. Mapping the opaque and holistic evolutionary way complex human biological systems of health promotion interact with the microbiome may require too much patience from bioengineers who are under pressure to produce not only results but profits. Has the HMP considered how the introduction of a genetically engineered microbe might influence or be influenced by both short- and long-term oscillations of the autonomic cardiovascular and immune systems, especially given the pervasive effects of modern stress?

Questioning the long-term consequences of meddling with germs is worthwhile because in the past medical science has underestimated grossly the long-term complexity of the relationship between germs and health. For example, the immediate success of penicillin in killing pathogens that had long been scourges of humankind overwhelmed consideration of longer-term evolutionary questions. Once antibiotic resistance presented itself, medicine followed the same formula in coming up with more potent antibiotics, effectively replicating in biology the cost arms race that medicine now finds itself in.

Prior to the discovery of the microbiome, no one was keeping an eye on the possibility that introducing extremely potent antibiotics could have an impact on the complex germ-IR balance by killing off health-promoting as well as pathological microbes, upsetting the microbiomic ecosystem. Thus no one knows the number or degree of health problems that antibiotic therapy may have precipitated inadvertently. The HMP has already found evidence for this unforeseen side effect of antibiotics on the microbiome, and one day soon the notion may gain the same boilerplate recognition currently accorded to warnings that inappropriate or excessive use of antibiotics may aid the evolution of antibiotic resistance in microbes.

$A''I$ offers a third direction for managing the microbiome that poses virtually no risk. Predictably, it is a poorly researched direction because all the attention and money flow toward bioengineering and diet (a multi-billion-dollar industry with well-defined markets). One recent study showed that a group of rugby players had healthier microbiomes than those of a sedentary group, suggesting that the autonomic cardiovascular and immune system effects of basic $A''I$ can shape microbiomic health (Reynolds). The effect of intermediate $A''I$ on the microbiome remains an open question, but given the stress-reducing, parasympathetic effects that intermediate $A''I$ has demonstrated, it too could promote a healthy microbial ecosystem.

The same can be said of advanced $A''I$. At this point, all I have is personal and anecdotal evidence along the lines of my pulsatile leap in Beijing. My biggest personal experience occurred while visiting a northeast coastal city in China during the late 1980's, where I picked up what seemed like a life-threatening gastrointestinal infection that I fought using the RfR. It took almost a week to subdue the vomiting and diarrhea, which became periodic abdominal pain for a couple of months thereafter, suggesting a persistent turf war between the invading germ and my microbiome. Since then, I have used the RfR to treat a number of less-hostile, food-borne gastrointestinal infections. By concentrating on the sense of falling, downward pressure of the RfR on exhalation, I have been able to dissipate quickly (in seconds) abdominal pain and discomfort and to promote the sensation of intestinal motility.

Such immediate control over disturbances in the microbiome indicate that sensing the RfR gives the RE practitioner control over the inflammatory chemical communications between gut-centered germs and the autonomic nervous system. Thus the constant experience of the pulsatile self may shape the microbiome to work with healthy oscillations of the autonomic cardiovascular and immune systems. Such a balanced IR can act as a positive evolutionary force on other microbiomes that work within the fabric of a vast interactive *macrobiome* of the environment. The condition of this complex give-and-take between the microbial worlds both inside and outside of the body elevates the importance of advanced A^uI and the cultivation of the pulsatile self through the RfR. Increasing the numbers of people who are able to maintain robust IR's would go a long way to promoting global health. It is an admittedly lofty and perhaps unrealistic expectation, but one well-worth considering.

Aging: The Final Complication

The majority of studies on the effects of aging on autonomic health show that over time the sympathetic rheostat gets turned up, probably because of diminishing vagal tone. This causes the kinds of imbalances induced by chronic stress. The loss of vagal responsiveness allows the upturned sympathetic rheostat to drive up levels of pro-inflammatory cytokines circulating in the blood stream. These higher concentrations of pro-inflammatory cytokines can produce an exaggerated pro-inflammatory response to infection. They also can disrupt the general function of the IR to keep the immune system oscillating between hot (inflamed) and cold (anti-inflamed).

One of the primary ways the IR maintains healthy oscillation is by identifying, weeding out, and replacing cells that have undergone *senescence*, a non-reproducing state that prevents a damaged cell from replicating. Once a cell becomes senescent, it expresses a "find-me" signal so that the IR can locate and eliminate it, and then summon up a replacement. The excessive pro-inflammation caused by aging probably dulls the IR's capacity not only to read the "find-me" signals, but also to call up replacements from stem cells residing in the bone marrow, lymphoid tissue, and fat deposits. With IR's elimination function impaired, senescent cells build up and further retard IR function. Multiple investigations have turned up links between excess senescent cells and several serious health problems in older populations, including Alzheimer Disease, heart disease, and cancer (Davalos, et al).

Immune effects, such as neutralizing a respiratory infection and routing its remnants to the surface of the skin, suggest that the RfR enhances the IR's ability to read the kinds of "find-me" signals produced by pathogens and senescent cells. As for the capacity to call up stem cell replacements, the evidence is considerably thinner. But one particular case shows there might be a stronger possibility than the evidence suggests.

After training in RE for about a month, a woman in her late thirties suffering from symptoms of early menopause acquired the RfR and consequently experienced an unusual side effect. She began spontaneously lactating, even though she had not breastfed her child for over two years. Moreover, she was taking high doses of estrogen, which, according to her doctor, should have repressed breast milk production.

Ordinarily it takes pregnancy and a cascade of hormones to spark lactation, but the IR also plays a part. During ordinary lactation, the mother's IR coaxes her body's most powerful lymphocytes out from the gastrointestinal glands and then directs those lymphocytes up into the milk ducts. Her IR then signals stem cells in the bone marrow to replace the reassigned troops. Those called-up stem cells transform into lymphocyte soldiers and make the long journey to their new glandular quarters in the gastrointestinal tract.

Both theory and research support the speculation that the RfR precipitated this case of mysterious lactation by reactivating the IR relationship between gut-centered lymphocytes, hormone-sensitive milk ducts, and the lymphocyte replacement function of stem cells in the bone marrow. If true, then one of the downstream benefits of cultivating the pulsatile self might be a heightened capacity of the IR to signal stem cells in the bone marrow and other tissues. Consequently, building the pulsatile self through persistent sensing of the RfR may prove to be an efficient and effective therapy to reduce the damages wrought by aging.

Chapter 9

Deeper $A''I$: Back-to-front RfR Circulation

Once the RfR has been experienced consistently over a period that typically ranges between three and six months, the RE practitioner can begin directing the RfR along a more complex and demanding pathway that runs up the back on inhalation and down the front on exhalation. The sensation of this RfR circuit initially is less pronounced than that of the frontal pathway, but over time it becomes more vivid, especially up the back pathway, along which a thick feeling of rising pressure appears to move. This deeper level of advanced $A''I$ extends the reach of the autonomic cardiovascular and immune systems and has a stronger impact on acute and overall health threats. In fact, this deeper level of practice has been essential in helping me subdue almost every health problem I have had over the past three decades, including the serious gastrointestinal illness mentioned in the previous chapter.

This deeper level of advanced $A''I$ has not yet been the specific focus of research, but a possible cardiovascular distinguisher emerged from the HRV study that compared seasoned RE practitioners with Mindfulness veterans. Almost all of the RE practitioners showed a sudden spike in blood pressure when they were told to start meditating, but a few sustained a level higher than that of the pre-meditation measurement throughout the meditation period, the sort of reading that might be caused by mild exercise involving movement. Those few were using the back-to-front pathway, suggesting that a mild, sustained increase in blood pressure distinguishes the back-to-front RfR circuit from a purely frontal circulation.

Because this was not a question the study was designed to answer, the finding was set aside. But the proposed theory of the neuro-biology of the RfR presented earlier provides and understanding of how and why back-to-front RfR circulation might cause such an effect. Mild blood pressure elevation indicates a dialed-up sympathetic rheostat, which means a greater volume of blood in the central artery through increased heart-rate, modulations in aortic diameter, or both. This greater volume of blood would push into and expand offshoots of the central arterial tree. With respect to back-to-front RfR circulation, the most significant of these vascular offshoots are the spinal arties, which project directly into the spinal column in six places, along with one projection into the brain stem near autonomic central. Increased central arterial pressure would inflate these narrow projections like balloons and push them into the spinal column space that contains cerebrospinal fluid (CSF), which is manufactured in the brain and flows down the spinal column into the lower spine, from where it circulates back up the spinal column into the brain in a cycle that is not well understood.

Illustration 30: Spinal Arteries Impinging the Spinal Column to Drive Circulation of CSF

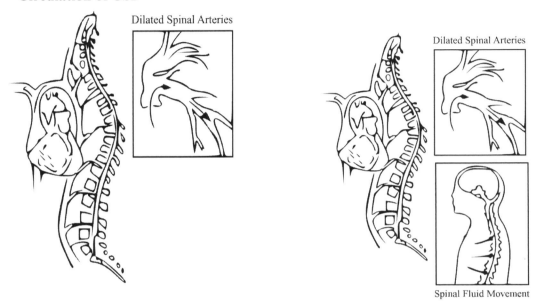

If the RfR sensitizes aortic barometric and chemical receptors as they respond to respiration, they could extend that sensitivity to sympathetic fibers lining the smooth arterial muscle to feel and control dilations and contractions of the spinal arteries and their influence on the CSF.

This possible effect is not mere speculation. In the 19th Century two British physicians named Monro and Kellie hypothesized that that mean arterial and CSF pressure have a strong positive correlation. That is, if pressure in the central artery increases, CSF pressure will increase as well. In other words, the autonomic cardiovascular system governs CSF circulation, thus making it *pulsatile*. The demonstrable effects of RfR circulation on HRV and BPV enhance the odds that cultivating the pulsatile self includes some influence over CSF pressure and circulation.

The Monro-Kellie hypothesis helps to explain how experiencing the RfR enabled veterans with m-TBI to reduce and even eliminate their chronic headaches, due in large part to sustained elevated cranial pressure. This increased cranial pressure indicates poor or stagnant CSF circulation and compromised flow within the blood vessels of the skull. Thus, when the veterans experienced the RfR, they may have been able to restore CSF and blood flow by modulating the autonomic cardiovascular system (and the autonomic immune system by default).

As mentioned previously, the discovery of the micro-lymphatic channels in the dural sinus cavity and nose provides an explanation for how the immune system breaches the blood-brain barrier. This obscure but important anatomical feature may hold the key to understanding how inflammatory diseases of the brain such as Alzheimer, Parkinson, and multiple sclerosis develop. It also surely plays a major role in the ability to sense and regulate the IR dimension of the pulsatile self, whether in directing the IR against an infection as I did during my pulsatile leap or in dampening and even arresting the inflammatory drivers of a disease with complex or unknown causes. This could be true even of some cancers.

Given these data points, it is reasonable to suppose that with back-to-front RfR circulation the RE practitioner can sense more deeply into this *cerebrovascular* system in order to promote CFS circulation, triggered by oscillatory dilations of the spinal arteries

Illustration 31: Theoretical Effects of RfR on CSF Circulation

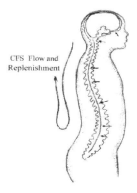

CFS Flow and Replenishment

and blood vessels that connect with the lymphatic tubules of the dural sinus and nose. Like enhancing the microbiome and stem cell production, this possibility bodes well for long-term health. CSF is the brain's lymphatic fluid, circulating important nutrients and immune-system chemicals filtered from the blood supply. CSF, micro-lymphatic channels, and the brain's venous networks also work together to remove waste from the brain. These functions require CSF circulation, as well as good blood flow, and so the ability to enhance CSF circulation should have a healthy impact on the brain.

There is another possible collateral health benefit that could result from regulating the autonomic cerebrovascular system. The brain uses up and remakes CSF between three and four times a day. Depleted CSF drains out of the brain and spinal cord through various structural apertures and ends up as waste in the lymphatic and cardiovascular systems, where the IR completes the elimination process. Like the cardiovascular and lymphatic systems, the CSF system is hydraulic, and so the drainage of depleted CSF most likely causes pressure-change signals that trigger the brain to manufacture more CSF.

But CSF replenishment also may rely on a chemical signaling process like that which the IR uses in replacing senescent lymphocytes. In fact, the new discovery of the micro-lymphatic channels of the dural sinus and nose makes this possibility a veritable certainty. By enhancing CSF circulation, back-to-front RfR circulation conceivably could

Illustration 32: Theoretical Effects of Back-to-front RfR Circulation on the IR

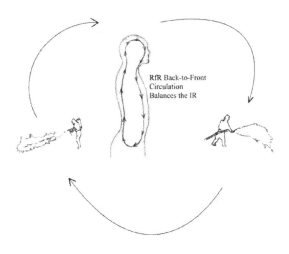

RfR Back-to-Front Circulation Balances the IR

exercise this pressure- and chemically-driven CSF restorative process, prompting the brain to keep the CSF fresh and strengthening the link between the IR and CSF elimination.

Deeper Still: Whole-body RfR Circulation

After practicing back-to-front RfR circulation from six months to a year, the RE practitioner can extend sensibility of the pulsatile self to the entire body. Like the other RfR pathways, whole-body circulation is driven by respiration and likely extends into the extremities the sensory connection between the aortic barometric and chemical receptors and the sympathetic fibers in the smooth-muscle lining of the arteries.

Whole-body RfR circulation begins with a deep exhalation and a falling sense of pressure down into the legs and feet. Then on inhalation, a mild pressure sensation rises from the heels, up the backs of the legs, into the tailbone, and up the spine where it concentrates around the seventh cervical vertebra. On exhalation, the pressure flows from the seventh cervical vertebra across the back and shoulders and down the backside of the arms into the backs of the hands and fingers. At this stage the sensation is more vivid, approaching the kind of thick quality felt during back-to-front circulation. Next, inhalation brings this more vivid sensation up the inside of the arms,   across the collar bones, into the larynx area, where the feeling rises up each side of the neck and joins a rising pressure sensation from the seventh cervical vertebra up the back of the head to the crown. With a final exhalation, the sensation falls along the frontal pathway, down the centerline that runs from face to torso, where it divides and passes into the front of the legs and continues to travel down into the feet where the cycle begins again.

The sensation of whole-body RfR circulation is far less dramatic than that of the frontal and back-to-front pathways, but its effect on pain and other inflammatory symptoms is remarkably fast and effective. For this claim there is no hard data. But over the years, I have had to use this more demanding form of RfR circulation to treat severe damage in my extremities.

The most recent occasion involved a knee injury I sustained when I tumbled head-over-heels down a flight of concrete stairs in an airport after returning sleep-deprived from a long business trip. It was after midnight, and I felt too exhausted to wait in an emergency

Illustration 33: Whole-body RfR Circulation—Initial Inhalation and Exhalation and Second Inhalation and Exhalation

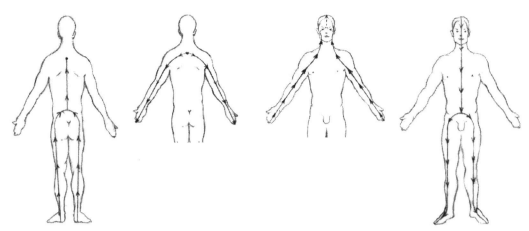

room to have a doctor tell me what I already knew was bad news, so I limped to my car and drove home. When I got there, my wife, who was over eight months pregnant, was sound asleep. It made no sense to have two miserable people, so I lay down on our living room couch and began doing whole-body circulation, with particular focus on my terribly swollen and painful kneecap. Each time the pressure-like sensation arrived at the injured knee, the pain would initially intensify and then diminish. Though I hardly slept at all, the self-treatment greatly reduced the pain.

The following morning, I wrapped an old ace bandage around my knee, dug through the closet for a pair of crutches, and drove myself to a prompt-care center. A technician took an x-ray, and the attending doctor examined the damage. She pressed around the knee area and shook her head. She said the x-ray showed that the kneecap was spit but that I wasn't presenting the kind of sensitivity to palpitation such an injury was supposed to cause. She recommended that I ice the knee and see an orthopedic doctor as soon as possible.

Because of serious athletic injuries I had sustained from martial arts and vigorous exercise over the years (a subject covered in the final chapters), I had a storied relationship with a University of Virginia orthopedist. The earliest appointment I could get was two days later, so in the interim I iced the injury, rested, and practiced whole-body circulation as much as possible. I walked into the orthopedist's office without crutches, and I when I stood using only the power of my legs to get up out of my chair to greet him, he expressed genuine surprise and then proceeded to show me why. On his monitor, he brought up the x-ray taken by the prompt care technician and showed me a gaping split in my kneecap. The good news was that the split was vertical, as opposed to horizontal, which would have meant surgically implanted screws and a far longer and more precarious rehabilitation. He advised me to wear a hinged knee brace for six to eight weeks and to spend as little time as possible on my feet.

Some advice I followed. I got and wore the knee brace, but I swam regularly and practiced daily whole-body RfR circulation during both a two-and-half minute Taiji routine and Seated Reflective Meditation. In three weeks, I dropped the brace. At six weeks, I was virtually back to normal, though I had to restrict the degree to which I could bend my knee. At my follow-up visit with the orthopedist, he shook his head and laughed, a concession that he was dealing with a medical anomaly.

Back-to-front and whole-body RfR circulation grows organically out of persistent, daily activation of the frontal RfR pathway, but both of these deeper levels of advanced $A''I$ require methods for honing and optimizing their efficacy. These methods are not taken up here but will be the subject of future research, as well as text and digital products that will be made available through www.pulsatileinternational.com. Nonetheless, awareness of these more sophisticated RfR circulations is an important aspect of understanding both advanced $A''I$ and the boundaries of the pulsatile self.

Unified Fitness: Integrating the $A''I$ Spectrum

As mentioned at the beginning of this book, all three levels of the $A''I$ build health by working the autonomic cardiovascular and immune systems. Basic $A''I$ helps to develop not only a broad range of desirable physical qualities—such as speed, strength, flexibility, agility, and attractiveness—but also a balance between the sympathetic and parasympathetic rheostats, so long as recovery, diet, and sleep are part of the package. Twenty minutes of running, swimming, or calisthenics spark the autonomic cardiovascular and immune systems, generating pulsatile, biochemical effects that can be sensed and more fully harnessed through a follow-on advanced $A''I$ routine like RE, which encompasses crucial elements of intermediate $A''I$. This integration of the $A''I$ spectrum provides a thorough means of working and establishing a sensory connection to the autonomic cardiovascular and immune systems. Meditation deepens the sensory connection so that the pulsatile self can exist more fully in non-meditative settings, such as downtime moments at work, lightweight chores requiring little concentration, travel, or even watching video.

This integration of the A^uI spectrum is called *Unified Fitness*, and if A^uI logic and the cumulative evidence have validity, it should be expected to provide superior control over autonomic health. In terms of basic A^uI, all that is needed is movement that gets the heart racing for twenty to thirty minutes, unless competitive athletics are involved, in which case health is less relevant and in fact may be in jeopardy. My own experience with rigorous exercise from childhood into middle age is that running and high-impact terrestrial sports are far more damaging to the body than is swimming, an opinion supported by a recent study that found that out of forty thousand men, those who swam for cardio exercise versus those who ran or walked suffered fifty percent less heart attacks (Chase, et al).

Far more important than athletic performance is following on with RE and working with the RfR, an emphasis that is likely to be resisted by those heavily invested in conventional fitness and athleticism. This investment in conventional fitness has health merits up to a point. But so far as autonomic health is concerned, conventional fitness has limits. Popular forms of intermediate A^uI such as yoga, "Tai Chi," and various meditative practices compensate to some degree, but they lack the capacity to awaken fully the sensory capacity of the autonomic nervous system and consequently the health benefits of experiencing the pulsatile self.

Unified Fitness offers a fairly simple method for building, maintaining, and controlling autonomic health that can be easily taught and widely distributed. If it were practiced on a global scale, humanity's power over health and disease would improve vastly, allowing conventional healthcare providers to focus on disease processes that are beyond the capacity of individual effort.

Part 3
The Origin of RE and the Limits of AuI

Chapter 10
The Grand Experiment

When modern China was founded in 1949, a grand public experiment in advanced A^uI was set silently in motion. In 1987—the year I made my pulsatile leap—the experiment was beginning to crest, and by 1989, it suffered the first of several blowups that would drive the possibility of open, widespread knowledge of the pulsatile self into obscurity, both within China and everywhere else. The history of this grand experiment is part of the legacy of advanced A^uI and is a tale that needs to be told.

Advanced A^uI knowledge resides only in cultures with long histories of looking inwardly for solutions to human problems. These inward-oriented cultures include China, India, Japan, and Korea (and neighbors subject to the gravitational influences of the big four). Of these four, only China escaped Western dominance. Instead, China was dominated from within by a native communist movement, led by Mao Zedong. This self-conquest and the reformation that followed had a unique impact on traditional culture, which in India, Japan, and Korea remained intact and competed with Western values introduced by British and American occupiers. In the case of communist China, Mao attempted to eradicate many aspects of traditional culture, especially religious superstition. But it appears that Mao or someone he trusted was willing to entertain the possibility of deeper mechanisms behind the superstition, because the government formed a number of Soviet-styled institutions to evaluate and reform traditional knowledge and methods, placed under the authority of cabinet Ministries. In the case of self-healing exercise, the Ministries of Health, Science and Technology, and Sport focused on their respective areas of expertise. Institutes under the Ministries of Health and of Science and Technology studied the effects that those accomplished in self-healing exercise were able to demonstrate. The Ministry of Sport concentrated on simplifying methods to produce large effects most quickly in order to enhance performance. The sport institute suited most naturally for this task was one of the historic incubators of self-healing exercise: the martial arts, which has a long historical entanglement with native Chinese religion and superstition.

Most experts agree that Chinese self-healing exercise originated in Daoism (Taoism), China's earliest indigenous religion, a form of nature worship that dates back four thousand years and is also the basis of traditional medical therapies such as acupuncture and herbalism. Daoism is also credited with founding a number of "internal" martial arts, such as Taijiquan, designed to use the soft-power principles of water to defeat those whose abilities relied solely on strength, hardness, and speed. Through a combination of movement and meditation, practitioners of these internal martial arts develop this water-like, soft power by cultivating *Qi*, or "vital energy," the Daoist universal "first cause," which permeates all matter and animates all living things. Daoists were the first to characterize health and illness in terms of Qi fluidity or lack thereof, a foundational precept of acupuncture. Health derives from the constant, unimpeded flow of Qi, while illness results from Qi disruption or stagnation. No one knows for sure, but one school of thought holds that the Daoists evolved this theory through the practice of self-healing exercise and the sensations it elicited. Some Daoists reputedly combined their self-healing practices with internal martial arts to the point where they could project their Qi as a telekinetic force that could destabilize, weaken, and even kill an opponent. Using Qi to fly, control natural forces, and live on eternally also stand out on the list of legendary bragging rights.

China's other famous traditional martial arts institution, a Buddhist sect known as Shaolin, applied the principle of Qi differently. Founded in the late 5th Century AD, Shaolin Buddhists developed martial arts routines and Buddhist meditations that reputedly foster extraordinary physical abilities, such as invulnerability to blows, swords, and spears, as well as exceptional strength and striking power. These powers were manifestations of greater vitality that lead not only to a longer mortal life, but also to enlightened control over the reincarnation process that Buddhism considers the ultimate concern.

Over the centuries, these two religious keepers of the martial-and-self-healing flame spread their knowledge (and their fantastic claims) to both high and low ends of the Chinese social spectrum. At the high end, Daoist and Buddhist knowledge holders transmitted their methods to aristocrats, elite physicians, academics, and military leaders, who shared a common education in the philosophy of Confucius, China's predominate cultural figure. This encouraged Daoist, Buddhist, and Confucian philosophies to converge around a number of principles, especially health and longevity, which became a core value of Chinese society as a whole.

At the low end, both Daoist and Buddhist monasteries would sometimes trade martial or health knowledge with villagers as a goodwill gesture or in exchange for food.

As a result, the martial and self-healing arts spread into and flourished in peasant villages, towns, and cities, where martial arts organizations formed and thrived across generations, sometimes basing themselves on religion and demanding supreme loyalty and commitment from their members.

In these ways, Daoist, Buddhist, and Confucian philosophy blended with spirituality, martial arts, self-healing exercise, and superstition to permeate all levels of Chinese society. Over the centuries this blend periodically spawned political turmoil, documented in both literary and historical texts. The opening of the Chinese classic *Romance of the Three Kingdoms* depicts a 1st-century Daoist uprising, which occurred again a century later. The wildly entertaining 13th-century novel *Outlaws of the Marsh* describes a small army of chivalrous martial artists and convivial murderers joining forces with Daoist and Buddhist monks to purge the monarchy of malicious imperial bureaucrats. As for actual insurgencies, in the 17th Century, when imperial power passed from the Ming to the Qing dynasty, the Shaolin Buddhists supported the Mings, and consequently were crushed by the victorious Qings. Reputedly, only five survived by fleeing into the wilderness, where they subsequently formed a martial arts insurgency and joined with other Ming loyalists to form the *Tian Di Hui* ("Heaven Earth Society"). In the 18th Century other anti-Qing militant groups organized, including one called *San He Hui* ("Three Harmonies Society"), which the colonial British translated into English as "the triad," a label that in the 19th and 20th Centuries became synonymous with Chinese organized crime.

Perhaps the most bizarre and catastrophic upheaval was the ironically named "*Taiping* (Heavenly Peace) Rebellion," initiated in the mid-19th Century by Hong Xiuquan, who formed his own version of fanatic Christianity after reading pamphlets written by missionaries. Driven largely by ethnic southern Chinese resentment over mistreatments by the northern Qings, the Taiping rebels held themselves together through a confused mixture of values that rejected traditional Daoist, Buddhist, and Confucian beliefs in favor of social parity, including separation of the sexes (even married couples) and sexual equality. Once they conquered a city, the rebels enforced their beliefs with extreme violence. In addition, a series of natural disasters that occurred over the fifteen years the rebellion lasted brought the death toll to an estimated twenty to thirty million, one of China's bloodiest uprisings on record. When the rebellion was finally crushed, remnants of the Taiping army fled to neighboring Indo-China or dispersed into the Chinese countryside and formed triads similar to those that arose in the previous century.

Given this track record, there should be little wonder why Mao decided to reform traditional martial arts and to purge them of superstition. To an extent, the plan worked. The state-run martial arts colleges not only simplified and formally reclassified overlapping and redundant styles that had evolved over the centuries of rivalry between religious sects and warring triads, but also refined and systematized self-healing exercise. A watershed moment in this process occurred shortly after Mao's takeover, when a scientist named Liu Guizhen classified all the myriad forms of self-healing exercise as *Qigong*, which translates as "Vital energy (Qi) skill (Gong)." Liu's name stuck and assisted in the mandate to simplify.

But the institutional extraction process was not entirely successful. Key traditional aspects were preserved that later would bring trouble. One such aspect was veneration of legacy. In the early years of Maoist reformation, claiming links to the past and to superstition was a mark of shame. But militant rejection of cultural history faded once Mao died, shortly after which the ban on Qigong was lifted. As Qigong began to make its way back into the public square, appreciation of legacy quickly resurged, suggesting a residual longing for the tradition that legacy rests upon: master worship, a core feature of Daoism, Buddhism, and Confucianism. Of the three traditions, Confucianism was most compatible with Maoism and thus was able to survive and to exert a stealth influence on family dynamics and the educational system through the central principle of elder and teacher veneration. Once Qigong became legitimate again, practitioners had an incentive to claim to have been taught techniques in secrecy by an elder relative or family friend who hid their powers following Mao's ban on superstition.

The other traditional aspect that made it through the refinement process was the concept of Qi, except that institutes under the Ministries of Health and Science and Technology re-imagined Qi in terms of Western atomic and biological science. They came to see Qi as a deep, energetic dimension of electromagnetic and gravitational forces that Western science somehow had missed. Increasing support rallied around this notion, which, enthusiasts trumpeted, ancient Chinese tradition had intuited and made legendary. Paranormal abilities such as extrasensory perception, telekinesis, and pyrokinesis studied by Western scientists operating on the fringe were recast as functions of Qi. This reinterpretation transformed Qigong into a new Chinese science that promised a means of understanding how to develop and to spread extraordinary powers throughout the citizenry. Manifestation of extraordinary powers became the first qualification for an authentic master. Having an impressive lineage ran a close second.

These two traditional traits of self-healing exercise dominated the grand experiment as it emerged from institutional sequester. Highly publicized accounts of skilled Qigong practitioners demonstrating *fa gong* ("projected skill")—the ability to use Qi as both a form of telekinesis and medical intervention, a legendary skill tied to Daoist and Buddhist superstition—seized both institutional and popular imagination. Projected skill involves emitting Qi from the body (primarily the fingers and hands) to move or destroy objects or to heal the sick, presumably through the same mechanism as that used by acupuncture. This external approach became known as *Wai Gong* (external skill), which overshadowed a self-directed approach referred to as *Nei Gong* ("internal skill"), pioneered by Daoist and Buddhist priests and their respective martial art cultures. The great appeal of *Wai Gong* as a therapy lay in the same kind of scalable advantage that acupuncture holds. With an army of highly-developed Qigong masters, whole hospital wards could be treated, requiring nothing more than passive cooperation from the sick, whose condition made learning a self-care exercise difficult.

One of the first Western records of the medical application of external Qigong was David Eisenberg's *Encounters with Qi*. A Harvard-trained physician who studied TCM in Beijing from 1979 to 1980, Eisenberg describes a Chinese doctor using projected skill to move a hand-made "dart" suspended in the air from a string and another using the method as anesthesia on a patient undergoing brain surgery. Teamed with journalist Bill Moyers in a follow-on to his book, Eisenberg returned to Beijing a decade or so later to film a PBS documentary of other seemingly miraculous demonstrations by Qigong masters. A particular standout was Shi Ming, a block-like, Mao-suited senior, who was shown making his students leap spastically into the air simply by touching them.

More sensational feats of Qi make Shi Ming's abilities seem fairly pedestrian. YouTube clips from the documentary *Ring of Fire* show Indonesian Qigong master and TCM doctor John Chang, or "Dynamo John" concentrating and waving his hand over a newspaper that subsequently catches on fire. More contemporary clips of other Qigong masters residing in the Far East show much the same.

The episodes Eisenberg recounts and the ongoing paranormal assertions made by master practitioners reflect developments documented in *Qigong Fever*, a detailed chronicle by David Palmer that tracks the rise of Qigong from relative obscurity in the early days of communist China to daily occurrences in public parks and eventually arena-rock-concert-sized crowds during the 1980's. Palmer's book corroborates that "projected skill" and master worship played an influential role in the spread of Qigong's popularity, but his account doesn't analyze historical causation, and it excludes evidence that projected skill and master worship were also instrumental in allowing some of the old socially destabilizing influence to grow. In essence, the grand experiment became another manifestation of the spiral of external solutions. It unsettled the secular socialist order by encouraging Qigong practitioners to interpret their experiences in ancient superstitious terms.

Maoist Masters in Deng's World

The societal shift that allowed Qigong to move from the institute into metropolitan China occurred when Deng Xiaoping took power in 1978. Palmer's chronology confirms that around that time classes began to be offered in Beijing's public parks, so the municipal and central governments either gave the go-ahead or looked the other way and let it happen. Thus a behavior absolutely forbidden in the previous decades began in the 1980's to gain popularity as means of shoring up public health. During this important epoch, hospitals began retrofitting with Qigong pre-existing Taijiquan programs established under Mao, who reputedly practiced Taijiquan because the benefits can be explained without mysticism. By mid-decade, Taijiquan and Qigong had become synonymous (sometimes referred to as *Taijigong*), because both involve coordination of breath with slow movement and the traditional concept of Qi. Eventually, Qigong evolved from a fringe practice used here and there as a legitimate intervention to a state-sponsored method of care, available as either voluntary public exercise programs or a form of medical therapy offered through clinics and hospitals.

Hospital and institutional backing legitimized and helped spread Qigong among the already considerably informed general public, many of whom had grandparents with a rudimentary knowledge of traditional medicine and Qigong. Deng's more liberal social policies effectively fertilized this social loam, out of which self-proclaimed Qigong masters sprang up like mushrooms in dark damp soil and accelerated the evolutionary process begun in the institutions. The traditional notion that Qigong masters were supposed to be elderly (as well as vigorous) was belied by young and middle-age hospital-based master therapists, who were sometimes physicians or paramedics with institutional accreditation. The competition that rose up out of the general population reflected this pattern, especially on college campuses, where Qigong found its most ardent support. There young Qigong adepts absorbed what they could from older teachers and read ancient classical texts preserved in libraries, and began experimenting with techniques to achieve more striking results. Supernatural lore sprang up around them. One of these young masters—Yan Xin, a professor at Qing Hua University whose rise and fall Palmer documents in *Qigong Fever*—claimed to be able to dematerialize and to heal lethal diseases from thousands of miles away. The government eventually would declare Yan Xin and other Qigong masters like him frauds, forcing them to flee to various regions of the West, where they continue to operate with far less luster.

The conditions that fostered such high enthusiasm for Qigong were well in place by the time I arrived at Beijing University, where well over a couple of thousand students, teachers, workers, and retirees practiced day and night. Similar sights could be seen on the campuses of the city's other major universities and colleges. Beijing University is China's Harvard, and so tends to attract the top talent in most things, and Qigong was no exception. There may have been fewer choices than what was going on outside the campus walls, but the quality was high, and translation was provided for foreigners who weren't there to learn Chinese. Within a six-week period, I met and trained with several Qigong masters, who displayed a bizarre combination of the historic forces that had wrought their methods. They used traditional concepts, but their methods and claims suggested institutional simplification and expedited results, enhanced by free-market competition. Some promised instant benefits, which stood in stark contrast to the traditional wisdom that progress came about slowly, a claim supported by all the books I had read on the subject and by the widely revered (at least in the U.S.) American kung-fu teacher I had studied with prior to moving to Beijing. In the rhetoric the 1980's Qigong masters used to recruit students, communist patriotism seemed to coexist comfortably with ancient tradition. Qigong was sold as a means to connect with China's rich cultural past and as a means to personal and national strength, thus making Qigong an inadvertent mouthpiece for the Chinese Communist Party.

The master I ended up studying with was cut from this cloth. For me, he seemed like the best choice because he was the head coach of the *wushu* (martial arts) team. But he also manifested the primary traits of a reformist Qigong master: young (in his late thirties) and patriotic, a former Red Guard who still very much loved Mao. He was dead serious about his mission and competed passionately against rival Qigong masters who trolled the campus in search of followers. His Chinese students got the best qualities of the modern Maoist master. He was wildly popular and virtually gave away his Qigong secrets as part of his patriotic duty to improve the health of his fellow citizens, who repaid him with devotion and service, which was about all they had to give. His charity had a practical side, too. Constant competition with other nationalistic masters who low-balled their rates and promised powers beyond mere health benefits forced him to do the same. His main rival, an even younger man with no martial arts abilities, boasted a class with over a thousand participants, twice the size of my teacher's largest class on campus (he ran other classes off campus). From time to time this master as well as other competitors dispatched spies to my teacher's classes to steal techniques, and on a couple of occasions he returned the favor. Several of these rival masters, including the one with the thousand-strong class, sent emissaries to my room to persuade me to defect, which gave me the opportunity to ask questions and find out the differences between my teacher's approach and theirs. These private Q&A's went on over the course of a couple of months without my teacher's knowledge until I was finally satisfied that I should stick with him.

What cinched my allegiance was my first experience with the RfR, which also gave me an existential basis for asking the recruiters of rival masters what was going on in their classes. The feedback I got was that they and their fellow students also were being taught to feel the RfR described in terms of Qi moving along acupuncture meridians. They also claimed to have developed the ability to move the sensation along the deeper circuits in a matter of months, sometimes weeks, an accomplishment unheard of by traditional estimates, which attribute such high-level abilities to at least ten years of slavish practice and a great deal of luck.

These students of Beijing University, as well as many students of other elite colleges and universities in Beijing, were experiencing the first-wave effects of China's institutionally accelerated grand experiment with Qigong. But these speedier results seemed to kindle rather than deflect Qigong's superstitious elements. In particular, government and popular support for external Qigong, with its emphasis on the supposedly superior capacity of the Qigong master to control Qi, encouraged Confucian, Daoist, and Buddhist superstition and master worship, which attributed powerful bodily effects such as the RfR to the master's Qi, not to that of the individual. The Qigong culture of Beijing in 1987 communicated almost entirely through these interpretations, placing the master squarely at the head of a congregation that received his emanation as though it were the Holy Spirit. In this manner, Qigong classes for public health effectively became a liturgical religion, promising extraordinary powers through the grace of a loving, traditional Qigong master. By comparison, the ability to cure the common cold through an internal sensation along the lines of the RfR was weak tea indeed, and so became hardly worth mentioning in the face of such fantastic possibilities. As a result, the RfR failed to register in both Chinese and outsider documentations of the rise of Qigong. Before clearer heads could prevail, the volatile social effects of traditional self-healing exercise began to assert themselves.

Both the spread and obfuscation of the RfR in the midst of the "Qigong Fever" that swept Beijing and other large cities in the 1980's is something for which the state-run martial arts college system deserves considerable credit. The most prestigious of these martial arts colleges—the Beijing Wushu Institute (BWI)—was only a short distance to the north of Beijing University. As a graduate of the BWI, my teacher had gotten direct access to that institution's collective wisdom when he was a standout athlete in the middle 1970's. One day he decided to take me on a tour of the place so that I could understand the value of what he was offering me.

The campus resembled those of all the other large colleges I had seen: at the main gate, a large statue of Mao, smiling and waving; a mixture of traditional and characterless Soviet-style buildings, spread out across grassless grounds, dotted with poplars and willows. We parked our bikes and went inside a large gym where I got my first peek at how the Maoist institution was cross-fertilizing Qigong and more traditional Western sports. While Olympic runners raced around a track, a few were seated on a bench in meditative postures, apparently circulating the RfR.

Next we walked across the way to a smaller gym where a gang of foreigners were learning a relatively elementary form of wushu. Two young teachers were putting the foreign students through their paces, correcting hands, stances, and facial expressions. My teacher walked over and began chatting with an older professor-coach, so I moved closer to watch the foreigners. When their coaches gave them a break, they roved over to check out the new guy. After I explained I was learning privately from my teacher, a few offered details of their own histories, most of which had to do with the lineage of their training in the West. When I asked them about the cost and extent of their stay in Beijing, all answered they had paid the BWI one thousand U.S. dollars in exchange for room, board, and a week's worth of training. None were being taught Qigong, nor were they especially interested in learning it. On the bike ride back to Beijing University, I expressed amazement that the foreigners were not being taught Qigong, to which my teacher responded proudly that now I had proof that I was getting a much better deal than I could possibly hope for.

My teacher never overtly credited the BWI for his Qigong methods. In fact, he presented his approach as a "system" he had inherited through his blood line, somewhere between three to five hundred years old. He called it "Three Emperors," essentially a martial arts triad founded on the Daoist divine trinity of "Heaven," "Human Being," and "Earth" (the "Three Emperors"), which correspond respectively to the three regions of the body—the head, the chest, and the pelvis—that are also the key "reflection sites" of the cardiovascular system. Qigong masters that my teacher competed with made similar claims about their methods, an expression of popular nostalgia for the comforts of China's venerable traditions. What I observed at the BWI suggests that innovation played a greater role. In retrospect, my teacher's system was likely an amalgam of techniques he had picked up from one of his relatives as child and from the BWI once he became a state-sponsored martial artist. His lineage to "Three Emperors" grounded him in the credibility of the ancient tradition, but his BWI training gave him the advantage of simplicity and producing quick results. He was doing instinctively what any businessman would do: delivering a superior service in order to beat the competition for foreign money, that is, the BWI. The only problem with his business plan was that the value of his best product—the RfR—was undervalued to the point of obscurity.

If "Qigong fever" obscured the RfR for Chinese practitioners, then it should come as no surprise that the tiny foreign cohort that sampled Qigong at that time was also kept in the dark. During the two years I lived in China, not a single Beijing foreign resident I met shared much interest in, much less my experience with the RfR. Only a few Westerners admitted practicing Qigong, which they did begrudgingly because a martial arts teacher had insisted. They talked about feeling their "Qi," having cosmic visions, or banging their hands and arms into trees or rocks, but no one mentioned anything resembling the RfR. The reason for this can be explained pretty simply. Either their masters didn't know the right technique or they knew the technique but withheld it from foreign eyes, a time-honored tradition in East Asian martial arts.

When asked about "extraordinary powers," contemporary masters, like those operating at the height of the "Qigong Fever" epoch, resort to TCM explanations that center on "preserving and cultivating Qi" and years of assiduous daily practice of a carefully guarded and highly prized method they earned by either birthright or devotion to a master teacher. In offering these explanations, these extraordinarily powerful (or perhaps fraudulent) Qigong masters demonstrate a kind of consistency that merits serious consideration and thorough investigation. But when these same masters have gotten serious enough consideration to have an investigation conducted, they have been unable to replicate their miraculous effects. The Qigong masters and their advocates retort that such Western-style investigations constitute a kind of anti-Qigong magic that undermines the deeper reality of Qi, which depends on trust and respect for the master. From the traditional Chinese perspective, master worship trumps scientific skepticism, an argument that renders Western scientific inquiry invalid.

The concept of $A''I$ provides one way around this apparent loggerhead. Instead of focusing on extraordinary powers, $A''I$ avoids the issue. But it also offers a tenable alternative explanation for extraordinary powers. Given that the autonomic nervous system is bioenergetic and linked to both consciousness and the sense of touch, it seems at least worth considering the possibility that ancient Chinese methods of self-care yoke together those biological faculties in some unique fashion that imparts the ability to project and effect fine sensory control over the immediate environment. This control could include the autonomic nervous systems of other people, which would explain Shi Ming's ability to make his students leap at his touch. Using such an explanation for pyrokinesis, levitation, and dematerialization, however, pushes things too far.

While such questions may be worthy of study, paranormal demonstrations and claims by Qigong masters have limited value compared to the practical benefits of advanced A^uI described in Part 2. If forced to choose, which would you rather have: the ability to set paper on fire or cure your own cancer? For the time being, Qigong practitioners who claim "extraordinary powers" are best viewed skeptically as outliers, along the lines of similar paranormalists all over the world throughout human history. Arguments that science is somehow inimical to Qi become irrelevant when controlling human health through known mechanisms is the focus of the question. A^uI works well with that focus because it is a concept that deals with phenomena that can be comprehended and tested by science.

Chapter 11
From Tiananmen to Falun Gong

Translation issues and traditional secrecy alone are not enough to explain why the Chinese Qigong authorities have never openly acknowledged the RfR. A deeper, far more complicated chain of events is to blame. The scope and scale of these events is so large and touches on so many other factors outside of Qigong that even to approach the topic invites controversy among experts in the West and many of the Chinese who were affected directly by the events themselves. Nonetheless, a discussion of these events helps account for how something so important and potentially world-changing has managed to escape recognition by the sharpest observers.

In much the same way 9-11 pulled all Western attention and resources toward Islamic extremism in the Middle East, the democratic focus of the Tiananmen Square protests of 1989 came to dominate all Western discussions of China, and it continues to do so. The rise of Qigong, inherently unintelligible to Western eyes, became an afterthought and finally irrelevant. But here's a modest proposal: the spread of Qigong among the students at Beijing University helped spark the Tiananmen protest, in the same way large Christian movements of the past have galvanized great wars and political upheavals. A clear example of this is the Great Awakening, the early colonial Protestant revival that provided the emotional common ground that later allowed scattered colonists and frontiersmen to come together to form the Revolutionary Army. In Beijing, from 1987 to 1989, a similar scenario played out on the city's major university campuses under the noses of the Chinese government. As a visiting English professor at Beijing University, I was in a good position to witness the socio-political alchemy of this cryptic spiritual movement.

Qigong Is Better Than LSD

In the winter of 1987, shortly after I felt the RfR, *China Sports*, one of the few English-language sports magazine in China at that time, accepted an article I wrote on my experience with Qigong. The title—"Qigong Is Better than Aspirin"—was a direct quote from my teacher, who jokingly made the comment after I described the miraculous elimination of my respiratory infection. Given what I believe is Qigong's complicity in fertilizing the 1989 Tiananmen student protest, a better title might have been "Qigong Is Better than LSD"

I say this because the 1989 Tiananmen student protest, aka the Democracy Movement, shares some basic similarities with the countercultural uprising on the campus of the University of California, Berkeley in the 1960's. Like their UC Berkeley counterparts, the Chinese students swept up in the Democracy Movement were privileged in comparison to their peers, extremely bright, idealistic, and in possession of what they believed was a new consciousness that could transform their world into a better, freer place. Hallucinogens and a vague appreciation for Eastern philosophy and Aboriginal spirituality were instrumental precursors for the Berkeley movement. Among the Tiananmen protesters of 1989, an uncounted cohort had at least two years of the Chinese equivalent of a revivalist experience: the widespread somatic "magic" of Daoist, Confucian, and Buddhist Qigong practices that were really more along the lines of what the 1960's Berkeley students yearned for. In some cases the effects of these ancient religious behaviors were just as intoxicating and hallucinogenic as LSD.

One aspect of 1980's Qigong practice that may have played a direct role in preparing the way for political rebellion was a phase known as *zi fa dong*, or "automatic movement," which consisted of practitioners, sometimes hundreds at a time, lapsing into trance-like states. During these trances, they would either quake and shiver spontaneously or behave in more passive, schizophrenic-like manner, such as plucking imaginary flowers or combing an invisible head of hair. Some sobbed uncontrollably, some rolled around on the floor or ground, and others practiced spontaneous *fa gong*, waving their hands around the distressed, who intermittently would grow passive in response to the supposed Qi emanating from their comforters' palms and fingers. Sometimes Qigong practitioners would go into these trances in public classes, so any Westerner willing to take an early morning walk could catch glimpses of this behavior, which, of course, seemed absurd, even crazed.

Even for a convert like me, automatic movement was repellant and difficult to accept, though it was fascinating to watch. At all of the classes I attended, the Qigong masters encouraged students to engage in this seemingly crazy behavior, the purpose of which was to release "stagnant" or "sick" Qi. Some masters used the Daoist explanation

Qigong Practitioners Experiencing Automatic Movement Trance

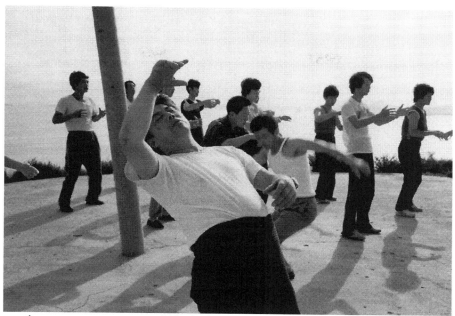

that automatic movement corrected "imbalances" between Yin and Yang, the primordial contrarieties that make up Qi. These imbalances explained the spontaneous use of "projected skill": the projectors supplied the half of the Yin/Yang that the recipient lacked or possessed in excess. Other interpretations relied on Confucian mysticism, claiming that entering automatic movement trances summoned ancestral spirits, which then took possession of the practitioner in order to drive out evil spirits or miasmas. Another common approach to explaining automatic movement was to fall back on Buddhism: the movements were a method of discovering and eliminating karmic snags or demonic entities lodged in the body. My teacher, as well as the other teachers I encountered, used all three explanations, as though they were interchangeable, in spite of contradictions or lapses in internal logic.

These religious interpretations of automatic movement lend credibility to the hypothesis that Beijing circa 1987 saw large numbers of Chinese turning back to remnants of native spiritual traditions, especially on the campuses of Beijing's major universities. But the automatic movement fad also sparked aberrant behavior outside of the Qigong class. Recurrent reports of Qigong students committing suicide or engaging in bizarre, socially unacceptable acts such as public nudity gave rise to an expression among the growing critics of Qigong: *zou huo ru mo*, translated as "walk fire, enter devil," a synonym for Qigong-induced madness, a development also recorded by Palmer in *Qigong Fever*.[+]

To head off these kinds of disturbed reactions to Qigong, masters at Beijing University implemented a custom that provided a rhetorical opportunity to decompress the emotion released during automatic movements. Following the physical catharsis of trances, students sometimes made public confessions or read out loud from diaries they were encouraged to keep, a practice that resembled the revered Maoist practice of self-criticism. The open confessions I witnessed took place in gymnasiums, and they combined magical descriptions with emotional content. Most significantly, students frequently included complaints about the limits of life in China, something that never would have appeared in a Maoist self-critical document. The masters sympathized with the students' hardships and lauded their honesty and candor, but never openly condoned disparagement of China's government and always topped things off with the advice to keep practicing Qigong in order to build the strength needed to work in unity for a "glorious socialist future with Chinese characteristics."

While the percentage of the student population exposed to these Qigong confessionals was difficult to pinpoint, their numbers went well beyond the fifteen hundred or so that made up the sum total of my teacher's and his chief rival's followers, because all were encouraged to "evangelize" on behalf of their masters and systems. At the time, I was too overwhelmed by the complexity and expansiveness of what I was seeing to understand I was in the midst of an evolving health cult with reciprocating religious and political traits. But from the multiple private conversations I had with the students caught up in this rapidly mutating society, there was little question that automatic movement and the group therapy sessions that followed were providing steady, repeated opportunities for the expression of compressed anger toward the status quo.

A more general source of release for bottled-up rage among both students and faculty was the expanded freedom of expression they enjoyed under Deng Xiaoping, whose policies were spring-like compared to the bitter winter of Maoism. Many professors who

---

[+] Both the Chinese medical community and the official Qigong authorities have used the expression for a variety of psychoses that have been observed in Qigong practitioners. The expression "automatic movement" has faded out of official Qigong rhetoric.

had survived the brutality of the Great Cultural Revolution despised communism and transmitted their feelings to students, a good number of whom had their own stories to add to those of their professors. Deng's policies also had exposed students and faculty on an unprecedented level to Western lifestyle and culture, which seemed like heaven in comparison to their own. Without the teeth of a rabid Maoist ideology that demonized the West, young educated Chinese responded to this exposure with dreams of escaping to luxury in the West, or even more fancifully, in a "democratically reformed" China. Consequently, students opted for one of two coping strategies: make a full-court press to migrate to the West (preferably the U.S.) or quietly and morbidly accept their limitations. In 1987, Qigong appeared to be giving students a way to make the likelihood of the second option more palatable.

In 1988, circumstances changed, and the impatience of the educated class with the government came increasingly into the open. One highly symbolic incident occurred in late April, when administrators at Beijing University, with the backing of allies in the Ministry of Education, arranged for two statues of Mao Zedong that stood in prominent places on campus to be dynamited. In front of the library, where Mao famously once worked and evolved a fuming contempt for intellectuals, a large crowd of faculty, students, and workers gathered to observe Mao's head chiseled off the large stone monument, which was then dynamited. Each group reacted with significant differences. Though far from gloating, the faculty and students' reactions ranged from modestly cheerful to stoically triumphant. The workers, who had been the intelligentsia's main persecutors under Mao, seemed both puzzled and hurt. As though to mock the Great Helmsman's 1950's "hundred flowers" campaign that was used to incriminate intellectuals, large beds of colorful tulips replaced the statutes.[*]

This incident was followed by another on May 4, when the University held its annual ceremony to commemorate the 1919 protest against Japanese occupation that gave rise to the Chinese Communist Party. Both students and faculty filled the campus movie theater where a series of speeches were to be held. Foreign teachers were allotted a row of

---

[*]The campaign got its "hundred flowers" name from a speech Mao gave in 1956, during which he encouraged criticism of his new government. Mao analogized this willingness to tolerate criticism to letting "a hundred flowers bloom." Soon thereafter, the "hundred flowers" campaign transformed into the "Anti-rightist" campaign, a forerunner of the Great Cultural Revolution.

choice seats in the middle. After polite but routine addresses by the president and a few other administrators, an official of the Party got up to give the final speech. Not more than a sentence or two into his speech students began booing and hissing, while the faculty and administration quietly looked on. The Party official's face reddened. Lowering his head, he struggled through at least ten solid minutes of open derision and interruption. Even the most experienced foreign teachers were horrified; they had never witnessed such blatant contempt for the Party. Scanning the faces in the crowd, I recognized a number of students who had been devout Qigong practitioners the previous year. One year later these former Qigong practitioners turned hecklers would be lost in the sea of student protestors who saturated Tiananmen Square.

If Qigong cults infused the cauldron of 1988 with volatile emotions, then action taken by the U.S. to tighten its China immigration policy near the end of February 1989 turned up the heat. News of the policy shift set off a student panic that one of their possible escape routes was being cut off. A stampede bore down on the visa office of the American Embassy, where by mid-March, the daily queue averaged a mile long, with many living on the street in order to preserve their places. In April, the flame under the cauldron got turned higher. Former Education Minister Hu Yaobang, who had been punished years earlier for openly calling for democratic reforms, died abruptly in a Beijing hospital. Because other politically liberal figures had died in similar fashion, rumors that Hu had been murdered exploded among faculty and students, who gathered in Tiananmen Square with wreaths and photographs to commemorate Hu, whom they characterized as a martyr for democratic reform. At first the gathering was small, but soon frustrated students living on the street outside the U.S. Embassy joined in. Within a month their numbers swelled and they articulated themselves into what became known as the Democracy Movement, which not only paralyzed Beijing, but spread throughout the country.

The shift in U.S. immigration policy and the death of Hu Yaobang were directly responsible for matters getting out of hand. But then without adequate animus, these two events may not have elicited such a vehement student response. The source of that student and teacher animus was deep-seated, connected to the abusive legacy of Mao and the protracted purges conducted over a thirty-year period. But from where I sat, student-based Qigong cults played a part in releasing and giving voice to that spirit, just as hallucinogenic

The Beginning of the Democracy Movement at Beijing University

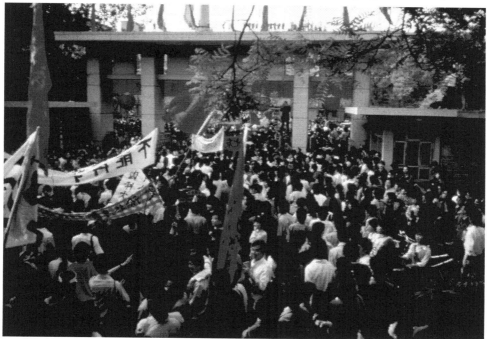

drugs and half-baked Far Eastern and Native American spirituality inspired the protesters on the campus of the University of California, Berkeley.

Aside from the reasons already cited, I stand by this hypothesis because Qigong cults generated such a powerful combination of hype and striking psychosomatic effects like the RfR. Migrating out of official greenhouses on the enterprising backs of people like my teacher, methods that produce the RfR became part of a host of triggering factors for the revival of superstition. Obscured by traditional rhetoric and the pressure to exaggerate in order to compete with methods promising supernatural powers, this extremely important subset of practices never registered in the inquiries conducted by Palmer and other Qigong documentarians. Adding to the obfuscation, my teacher as well as every other teacher of the Qigong community I was exposed to would have denied any innovation on their part, because antiquity had, and still has, great weight in Qigong culture.

In discussions with various China experts about the validity of the Qigong-Tiananmen hypothesis, I have been asked routinely for corroborating testimony from others who were present at the time. As I've already stated, no other foreigners to my knowledge were willing to participate to a deep enough extent in Qigong and therefore could not have taken in the details I witnessed firsthand. Chinese Qigong practitioners, bound by traditional interpretation, lack the objectivity to perceive a cause-effect link. Moreover, a surviving protestor who agrees that Qigong may have contributed to Tiananmen might risk criminal liability if living in China or banishment if living abroad. Student and senior intellectual leaders who became celebrity causes for Westerners outraged by the government crackdown aren't likely to consider a Qigong connection to the Democracy Movement because doing so could detract from the rational motives behind the uprising.

Finally, Chinese officials are unwilling to admit a Qigong-Tiananmen link for several interconnected reasons. First, the government would prefer to never talk about Tiananmen because it is a source of shame and embarrassment. Second, a government admission that Qigong contributed to Tiananmen would make the government, i.e., Deng Xiaoping, complicit in the matter since it/he allowed and even encouraged Qigong culture to flourish prior to the Democracy Movement. Third, the government has solid evidence that Qigong has a tremendous public health potential and as a remnant of ancient Chinese culture deserves to be esteemed and preserved, not vilified as a bringer of social chaos.

One thing I am sure of is that the Party was in the loop on what went on in those Qigong therapy sessions at Beijing University. A young man the Party assigned to shadow me was present multiple times when these confessions took place, and I have little doubt that he ended up making a thorough report to his superiors. Under these circumstances, it seems likely that at the very least the Party has considered connecting these dots.

Chapter 12
Falun Gong: Tiananmen 2.0

A crucial event that sheds some light on the possibility that the Chinese government suspects a Qigong-Tiananmen link is the government's reaction to the 1999 May protest in Tiananmen Square by followers of Falun Gong, the biggest Qigong cult in China's modern history. The Western consensus on the crackdown is that it was a paranoid overreaction to what Falun Gong advocate David Owenby points out began as a sit-in conducted in the eastern city of Tianjin by a relatively small group of elderly women. When word spread that the Chinese police were dragging away these grannies, the Falun Gongers responded in force. Though there is no official headcount to my knowledge, a group reported to be as large as ten thousand showed up at Tiananmen Square to stage a protest. The government's response was swift and brutal, and it didn't stop once the protesters cleared the Square. Falun Gongers were thereafter imprisoned, tortured, and censured until the only objections heard were those from supporters and sympathizers outside of China. There can be little question that Falun Gong's ability to forge trans-regional and trans-class alliances without the government's becoming aware spooked the leadership. Aside from its own organizational talent before 1949, the Chinese Communist Party hadn't witnessed such an immediate demonstration of people power since the Democracy protest of 1989.

The Falun Gong demonstration's eerie similarity to the 1989 student protest nightmare undoubtedly distressed the central government, especially because it had made considerable effort to regulate Qigong after the 1989 Tiananmen crackdown. Initiated within the Ministry of Health, those regulatory efforts took a significant turn in the mid-1990's, when the task migrated to General Wu Shaozu in the Ministry of Sport. This reassignment of responsibility suggests the government's intent to convert public perception of Qigong from a mystical practice to a physical mind-body exercise, just as the collegiate system had done with martial arts. Wu's regulatory approach resembled the way the Federal Food and Drug Administration controls the pharmaceutical industry. As Palmer notes in *Qigong Fever*, such formal regulation partially existed prior to Tiananmen, but Wu's policy was the most comprehensive to date, and its effect was to greatly restrict the number of Qigong systems that were allowed to compete, thus limiting cryptic religious freedom that had cropped up inadvertently under Deng's liberal hand.

By the mid 1990's, Wu's team had recruited Qigong masters it felt were reliable and effective (following the BWI model of the 1950's) to staff the China National Qigong Institute (CNQI), whose role was to help formulate Qigong accreditation criteria. These criteria emphasized demonstrable proof, but they also put China's cultural stance toward Qigong on equal footing with that of Western science. As a result the magical properties of Qi once again were preserved. While probably a manifestation of China's desire to create an exclusively Chinese science, this continuation of the traditional mystification of Qi opened a doorway to trouble with Falun Gong.

In his book *Falun Gong*, founder Li Hongzhi lays out his system in terms that follow guidelines created under Minister Wu. Li uses ancient cultural tropes, but also interlaces selective concepts of Western atomic science to explain Qi and the miracles he was able to accomplish with it. These explanations and the actual exercise don't radically depart from those of other systems which Falun Gong competed with for attention and membership. The breathing technique, some of the movements, and meditative postures resemble those of the system I learned and others like it, which I believe migrated out of institutes like the BWI via my teacher and others like him. Thus Falun Gong may have enabled many of its devotees to feel at least vestiges of the RfR, but more importantly its presentation hit the sweet spot for many Chinese. The defining symbol Li chose for his system was the *Falun*, or "the Great Law Wheel," depicted as a Tibetan Buddhist swastika, flanked in its quadrants by four Daoist *Taiji Tu* (Yin/Yang diagrams). According to Li's book, practicing his routine allows the practitioner to *sense* (a key word) the Great Law Wheel in the lower abdomen, the region traditional Qigong refers to as *dan tian*, typically translated as "field of elixir," the source of the RfR's interoceptive pulse sensation that is at the heart of the method distilled in the Maoist institutional greenhouses. As Owenby, Palmer, and others have argued, Li's rhetoric provided a grand spiritual and social gloss that many post-Mao Chinese longed for: without proper social and spiritual growth all other effects of Qigong are trivial or delusional—not that much different from what most Qigong teachers were saying in 1987. The difference between Li's message and that of pre-Tiananmen Qigong culture is that pre-Tiananmen masters infused their spirituality with nationalistic pride and purpose. In *Falun Gong*, Li declares himself an update of Buddha, Laozi, Confucius, and Jesus Christ, creating an aura of inerrancy that his followers seemed willing to take seriously. This sort of boast brings to mind the kind of thinking behind the Taiping Rebellion, whose founder believed he was the long-lost brother of Jesus Christ.

The omission of secular patriotism in Falun Gong's spiritual rationale certainly didn't help its relationship with the government. On top of that, Li's actions and those of his followers when they butted heads with China's leadership worsened matters. Li left the country, and in his absence, those in charge responded defiantly to Wu's and the CNQI's insistence on experimental proof of efficacy in order to receive accreditation. This provoked the leadership and the officials under its direction to go on the offensive by disputing Li's spiritual autobiography. Like Yan Xin who preceded him in mythic popularity, Li claims to have been taught Qigong at an early age by a handful of religious masters, who transmitted to him supernatural powers that he kept secret during the Cultural Revolution. He further claims that throughout the 1980's he extensively "tested" his modified system, which he publicly launched at a Chinese middle school in 1992. According to Owenby, Chinese officials contend that Li lifted several of his methods from two other well-documented Qigong systems and a traditional dance routine he picked up while visiting relatives in Thailand.

The government's objection to Falun Gong on the grounds of authenticity appears disingenuous, since Li admits to a certain amount of creativity. And the organization's apparent reluctance to submit to experimentation doesn't supply a completely satisfying answer. More than likely, what upset the authorities was the gargantuan size of Falun Gong's membership and the organizational power it demonstrated in May 1999. Just before the ban on Falun Gong, the Ministry of Sport estimated that approximately sixty million citizens were practicing Qigong, making it the most popular form of exercise on the planet. Falun Gong's estimated ten million practitioners constituted a substantial portion of the Qigong market, giving unacceptable power to Falun Gong and Li. Adding to the government's worries, Li decided to venture abroad, which created the opportunity for another Tibet-like situation to develop, with Li acting as Falun Gong's Dali Lama, positioned to whip up sympathy in the West and to hand China's political enemies the means to impugn and harass. Thus, to the leadership it may have seemed better to take a world-opinion beating in the short run while a degree of control lay within reach: a lesson learned from Tiananmen. In time the matter would fade into irrelevancy, as other, more compelling issues captured the West's attention. China's economic rise has served that end.

Falun Gong's size factored into another social issue the Chinese government must constantly struggle with. China has a tremendous number of "migrant workers," a nicer way to say "homeless." In 2011, China's National Bureau of Statistics estimated the number of migrant-worker/homeless at over two hundred fifty million, over two-thirds of the entire U.S. population ("Statistical Communiqué on the 2011 National Economic and Social Development"). Imagine those numbers—hungry, disillusioned, angry— responding to historical, politico-religious impulses orchestrated by a spiritual leader who says he can control the weather (not a joke—Li claims to have done this) as well as provide health and happiness for all.

The big question is whether or not Tiananmen factored into the trifecta of Falun Gong's size, China's enormous homeless population, and historic precedence of Qigong-centered insurrections to provoke such a strong response from the Chinese government. If it didn't, based on what I saw happen during my two years on Beijing University's campus, it probably should have. Li's system appears to have embodied many of the qualities of the Qigong systems that captured the imagination of so many within Beijing's centers of higher education. Falun Gong is innovative; it emerged out of the competitive rigors of the 1980's; its rhetoric and reported effects suggest a blending of Mao-era simplification and traditional religious Qigong; it included Western science largely as a metaphor to explain itself, but ultimately settled on selective Confucian-Daoist-Buddhist principles for justification. Thus, the 1999 Tiananmen Falun Gong protest may very well have represented a second generation of what got obscured in the whiplash of the Democracy Movement's sudden rise and fall: a Qigong insurrection 2.0 to 1989's 1.0.

Two key differences between the Tiananmen and Falun Gong protests stand out. One, Falun Gong was not a youth movement; its membership cut across multiple demographic categories. In this respect, the relationship between the pre-Tiananmen Qigong and Falun Gong movements resembles the relationship between the UC Berkeley protests and the mainstreaming of counterculture a decade later. Second, unlike the student protest of 1989, the 1999 demonstration had its spiritual hunger out in full view, unencumbered by secular demands. Thus, what appeared to Western eyes a reaction that was excessive and paranoid may have been an over-correction for failing to understand fully the spiritual mechanics involved in Qigong culture that preceded the events leading up to the Democracy Movement. Unlike mainstream counterculture, which in the West quickly became another consumer market, the mainstream effect that Falun Gong had on Qigong led to defiance of the central government and thus posed a potential threat to the Party's hold on power.

Post-Falun: Qigong 1.5

In September 2007, Chinese officials responsible for Qigong management invited me to Beijing to present my ideas on RE and the RfR. During the visit, I marked a number of changes that had occurred since the Falun Gong crackdown. The Ministry of Sport still presided over Qigong matters, but General Wu had retired shortly after the Falun Gong protest, for which he was quietly blamed. The CNQI had been replaced by the Chinese Qigong Association (CQA), a panel of six that presented pamphlets, books, and DVD's of five officially-approved "Wellness Qigong" systems. There was no mention of the Qigong I had been exposed to in the free-market environment of the late 1980's. The "automatic movement" craze and the widespread practice of *fa gong* were also absent from the discussion. I asked why "opening meridians" was missing from their explanations of Qigong. After startled looks around the table, one of the CQA leaders—a dead-serious man with a silver crew cut—gave the uneasy response that "there are some problems with that form of Qigong." A bit more probing revealed that the form of Qigong that made the grand experiment so promising had been put back into institutional isolation. Only traditional doctors, professional martial artists, elite athletes, and special branches of the military were permitted officially to practice those methods.

As I packed up the new Qigong materials, disappointment clouded my thoughts. The grand experiment I saw in 1987, when so many Beijingers soared on the wings of transcendental interpretations of the RfR and its ancillary effects, had faded to obscurity, and an open discussion now seemed impossible. That sense of remorse overshadowed the spectacular transformation Beijing had undergone since the late 1980's. The neighborhoods surrounding Beijing University that once consisted of single-story buildings with traditional tiled roofs were gone, replaced by gaudy modern office towers, illuminated

2007 Meeting with CQA, the Author, and Dr. Tyvin Rich of the University of Virginia

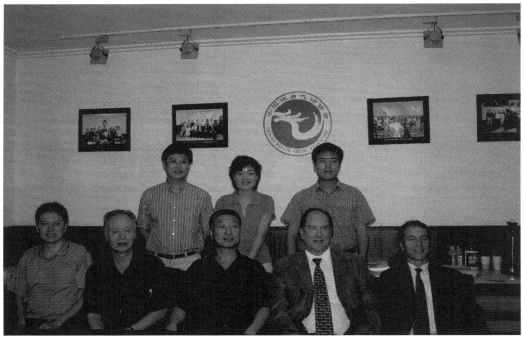

everything I had learned over the past twenty years about the rise and fall of the grand experiment. My former teacher had moved to Canada. The students had been militarized, forced to rise early and participate in an ROTC-like program to insure loyalty to the State. The building where I first experienced the RfR—at that time the best accommodation on campus—had been gutted. Across from the north wall of the University, on the once desolate grounds of the Imperial Garden where I had skulked about in the predawn darkness, mesmerized by the black shapes moving slowly in the cold air, palatial homes were being built.

My mood lifted when I was escorted to the Sports University, almost unrecognizable, with its gleaming new buildings and ornamental plants worthy of an exclusive liberal arts college of northern California. The BWI had also been upgraded to a cluster of new buildings embossed with both traditional and modern wushu statuary. I met briefly with the president of the Sports University and director of the BWI, whom I knew and had worked with previously. Around the time of the Falun Gong crackdown, I had hosted him and another BWI professor for several months, during which time I learned that they, like my former teacher, had honed their Qigong skill through the BWI.

After briefly discussing my fledgling research on RE, we toured of the facilities where the Olympic athletes trained. Not a penny had been spared in outfitting the athletes with the latest gadgets of Western exercise physiology, nothing like the Spartan conditions I had seen back in 1987.

Finally, we got to the real purpose of our visit: a meeting with the BWI's most venerated Qigong master, a man somewhere in his late sixties who had reputedly cured himself of terminal cancer with Qigong. The elder master wore the standard BWI workout uniform—t-shirt with nylon jogging pants—and his face was scarred and discolored on one side. His body was far more muscular and fit than that of other athletic men his age I have known, but its odd stiff angles and alignments showed he had paid the price of doing martial arts for a living. We followed him into conference room, sipped mugs of tea, and had a lengthy discussion mediated by translators. The discussion vacillated between polite chit-chat and serious questions that eventually made clear the master's Qigong system fit the wellness paradigm of the CQA, with a particular emphasis on the traditional explanation that his system produced good health by enhancing Qi flow, which ultimately was reflected in an overall sense of contentment. After I stopped questioning, the master asked me how I had come to learn Qigong. I explained that I had learned from a BWI graduate back in the 1980's and had gained the ability to manipulate sensation along acupuncture meridians. An expression of mild disturbance I had learned to recognize during my two years at Beijing University momentarily registered on his face. He asked for my former teacher's name, and when I gave it, his facial expression resumed its former stoicism. "I remember him," the master said curtly. "He was pretty good." From a BWI professor of the master's status, this was high praise.

Before I left, I cornered the elder master's top foreign student, a beefy long-haired Frenchman, who was in the process of sheathing a Taiji sword. I asked him how long he had been practicing wushu, and he said he first trained at the BWI in 1986 and that he had a large Taiji and Qigong following all over France and parts of Europe. I mentioned that I had been at Beijing University from 1987 to 1989, and we laughed that we had probably seen each other.

"What do you feel when you practice Qigong?" I asked.

He looked off into space and said the elder master's method was to search the mind for troubling thoughts and then classify them according their association with particular organs.

"For example," he said. "I may feel some anger, which unbalances the liver, so I do my Qigong exercises and direct Qi to my liver to correct the imbalance."

"Do you ever feel a pulse that you can move up and down the body?"

"No," he said, puzzled. "It's just as I described."

We shook hands and departed. When I rejoined the others in my group, I asked the BWI director if the Frenchman could sense and control the "Small Universe," the traditional name for back-to-front circulation of the RfR.

"No," he said.

"You mean after so many years, he still hasn't been taught?"

"I don't think so."

Throughout the remainder of our stay in Beijing I brooded over the ramifications of our meetings with the CQA and what I had learned from the elder master's French disciple, who clearly had gotten caught in China's early official approach to capitalizing on foreign interest in wushu and Qigong without revealing the secret. Given the chaos Qigong had proven it could elicit, perhaps what we were being shown was the best that could be done for the time being. One thing was certain: what I had seen and gotten from my time in Beijing was long gone.

To get a feel for how things were playing out among the natives, the following morning I paid a visit to the Temple of Heaven in the heart of Beijing. There in plain view was what the casual observer might consider the same sorts of things I had seen in 1987. Thousands of Chinese of all ages—though most were middle-age and elderly—exercised in some form or fashion, from ballroom dancing and jogging to Taiji and official Qigong. One group stood around and did nothing but smile and giggle, so-called "Laughing Qigong," the latest Wellness Qigong craze. But as I ventured further into the park, I saw elderly men doing old wushu forms. One man in particular caught my eye because of his well-defined musculature and crisp movement. After completing a fast routine, he began moving in ways I recognized as having the potential to effect the RfR. I waited for him to finish, then asked him if he could feel his Qi moving along the traditional Chinese equivalent of back-to-front and whole-body RfR circulation. He smiled proudly and nodded.

That 2007 visit to China led me to four conclusions. First, the form of Qigong I initially learned most likely owed its efficacy to institutions like the BWI. Second, Falun Gong and other similar systems possess elements that can produce at least vestiges of the RfR. Third, the ability to sense and build the pulsatile self through the RfR is probably widespread among the population of China's larger cities, but those who have the ability have gotten the message not to publicize their ability or to teach for fear of being associated with Falun Gong or similar outlawed Qigong cults.

My fourth conclusion is that it was no fluke that a highly accomplished martial artist and Sinophile like the French disciple of the elder master was ignorant of the RfR. The attention-grabbing power of traditional master worship and the super-scientific properties of Qi proved as irresistible to foreign converts as it was to native Chinese. Consequently, Western Qigong converts like the Frenchman ended up serving as vectors for transporting considerable hype from the grand experiment to the relatively pint-sized, diffuse alternative-health culture in the West. By and large, the hype, which requires buy-in to traditional Chinese tropes, proved a tough sell in a very small marketplace with tight margins, already filled with the hype of rival methods that had gotten to the Western chalkboard first. As a result, Western Qigong converts have done little more than to introduce exercises that function at basic and intermediate A^nI levels.

Chapter 13
The Limits of A^uI

China's grand experiment provides a cautionary tale for the limits of A^uI. Born of an inwardly directed culture with an ancient tradition of advanced A^uI, the grand experiment got hijacked by the deeply human need to experience the fantastic. This hyperbolic tendency is a higher brain function intrinsic to imagination, spirituality, and most likely the HPE. It allows us to see and become inspired by greater possibilities, ideas, visions, or dreams that lead to progress, or, as was the case with China's grand experiment, delusional thinking and social disorder. In all cases, imagination is interdependent with the autonomic nervous system and can enliven or degrade its oscillations. This autonomic interdependence makes imagination a fourth meta-level on the A^uI spectrum. This fourth meta-A^uI level represents, in the priceless words of former Secretary of Defense Donald Rumsfeld, the realm of "known and unknown unknowns."

Figure 4
The Fourth Level of the A^uI

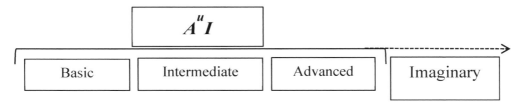

Anyone persuaded by the benefits of methods that function within the more knowable boundaries of basic, intermediate, and advanced A^uI can jump to this fourth-level playground whenever the spirit moves. The availability of effective advanced A^uI methods in inwardly directed cultures like that of China makes for a shorter jump to the fourth level. Lacking a deep culture of advanced A^uI, Westerners have to hop from basic and intermediate A^uI methods to imagination over a greater stretch of the spectrum. Visiting this playground is as easy and natural as daydreaming, regardless of cultural background. But when the visit goes on too long, the playground can turn into a trap. Megalomaniacal Qigong masters who believe they are superior incarnations of Buddha, vain fitness fanatics who over-train themselves into injury, self-absorbed meditators who fool themselves into thinking they are "enlightened," delusional energy therapists who believe they are egoless conductors of celestial powers but are really purveyors of false hope: all tarry too long at the imaginary A^uI level. Like the Greek mythological character Icarus, who used wax-coated wings to escape imprisonment, these fourth-level A^uI malingerers fly too far from the grounding principles of the A^uI spectrum, melt their wings by soaring too close to the sun of imagination, and plunge into an ocean of chaotic consequences.

From King of the Hill to King of Pain

My own Icarian flights of fancy beyond all three levels of the A^uI spectrum illustrate more specifically and pertinently than China's grand experiment the danger of imaginary A^uI. My childhood and adolescence were spent in slavish devotion to Western sports and physical fitness. In my late teens, I picked up East Asian martial arts that were more basic than intermediate A^uI but nonetheless opened me up to the possibility of contemplative practice. In my twenties, I turned my cumulative basic and intermediate A^uI skills into a private religion. The benefits of those skills strengthened my sense that I had found an unassailable fortress against the looming possibility of illness, loneliness, and premature death. I believed so completely in this private religion that I was unable to stop exercising after breaking my wrist while cycling and might have lost the use of my right hand had I not had the good fortune to be one of the few Westerners to go deep into China's grand experiment. Advanced A^uI knowledge enabled me to self-heal my wrist and control inflammatory symptoms, but it also inflated an already overblown sense of invulnerability, setting the stage for a series of personal catastrophes that would make my body a proving ground for the spiral of externality.

The set-up for misery began when I started a martial arts studio after returning to the U.S. in 1989. The program I created followed the Chinese tradition of using martial arts training as a way for customers to earn the privilege of being "let in" to my teacher's traditional "Three Emperors" Qigong method. Japanese and Korean martial techniques that were in my wheelhouse before my pulsatile leap were also part of the curriculum, but the centerpiece was Chinese wushu.

With the possible exception of gymnastics, wushu is the most exquisitely punishing form of basic A^uI there is. It demands moving full-tilt back and forth between low and high stances, as though in a sprint, putting tremendous pressure on the lower back, hips, knees, and ankles. It requires repeatedly launching the body into the air like either a Frisbee or arrow, kicking and punching simultaneously, even after coming out of a full forward flip. Wushu twists and extends the body in every conceivable direction, exhausting muscles and nerves so that by the time the exertion ends, the body wrings with sweat and the legs barely can manage walking straight.

The intermediate and advanced $A"I$ effects of Three Emperors Qigong and Taijiquan aided in recovery from this extreme exercise, which created the impression that I had established a well-balanced, health-promoting system in the traditional image of Chinese martial arts. But the system carried the same problematic elements that upended the grand experiment. With no credible scientific theory to account for the RfR, traditional explanations distilled from my teacher and other Qigong masters accounted for student progress and failure. The major premise of these traditional explanations was the Confucian rule that the teacher is the primary source of a student's ability to feel Qi rising and falling from lower abdomen to head. Getting the sensation meant the student had practiced according to prescription and earnestly venerated the teacher, the true source of Qi for the uninitiated. Failure to get the sensation indicated faulty practice, insufficient veneration of the teacher, or both. Under these conditions, the little society that grew within the martial arts school became divided and emotionally turbulent, which, as the school's master-teacher, I had the unpleasant task of dealing with. At the same time I constantly had to prove myself worthy of veneration. I demonstrated this worthiness not only by using "projected skill" to initiate what I referred to loosely at that time as "the pulse" in students during meditation, but also by maintaining exceptional health and strength. The main way I manifested this was by performing daily the most difficult wushu routines at a level superior to that of much younger students, many of whom became quite accomplished. It was no small matter of pride that at up until age forty-two—two years past the traditionally prescribed BWI retirement limit for athletic wushu—I could outdo even the best of the teens and twentysomethings I trained. These conditions, along with a sincere belief that the pulsatile effect I had obtained from Qigong could benefit humanity, combined to make me the de facto head of a health cult.

U.S. Wushu Teacher and Qigong Cult Leader

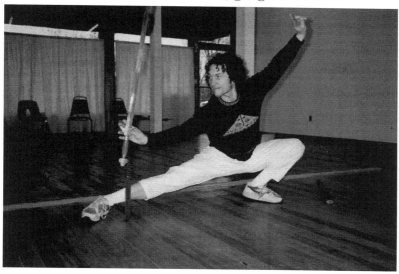

For seven years, even as I grew disenchanted with traditional Chinese explanations for Qi, dropped the dicey and unnecessary practice of using "projected skill," and began evolving toward the concept of $A''I$, I played the part with mixed feelings. On the one hand, my ego thrived over being king of my own little hill, a wellness guru and hotshot martial artist with a college professor's gift of gab that was attractive to enough customers so that I was able to pay the bills. But over this same seven years my life moved in an increasingly conventional direction. I married, fathered children, divorced, began a new relationship, and rediscovered the Christian faith of my childhood—all of which cast a pall of responsibility and limitation over my position as guru. My divorce deeply divided the already divided little society that evolved. Some quit in protest and affiliated with rival martial art and alternative-health teachers who were ignorant of "the pulse," enhancing the perception that there was nothing exceptional about what I was offering. This happened simultaneously with a growing determination to be taken seriously by important people with either medical credentials or money and power. I became so preoccupied with these and other relatively petty concerns that I ignored the possibility of taking a nasty tumble down my little hill and breaking something far worse than a wrist bone.

And then it happened, starting with a perfect storm of what seemed at the time a couple of small injuries. One day while trying to move one end of a three-hundred-pound trampoline I used to teach flips, I felt an odd tug in my lower back that resolved in a couple of hours but then became a bizarre soreness in my right leg whenever I lifted my knee above waist level. An hour or so later, I sparred with a large, aggressive student who landed a spinning side kick that felt as though it had caved in my right ribcage. Another hour later, it was time to put through their paces my most advanced wushu students, a pack of physically fit young teens who used my wushu performance as a benchmark. Determined not to show weakness, I led with the usual intensity, capping things off as I did everyday with an exhibition of the most difficult wushu form in the school repertoire, a two-minute routine put together by the BWI during the 1970's that was the equivalent of an eight-hundred-eighty-yard sprint, only with leaps, flips, and strenuously low stances. Though my entire right side felt as though it were being cleaved from my body, I completed the form without error. After twenty minutes of back-to-front pulsatile circulation, I felt better, but there was still another two hours of instruction to go before it was time to call it a day. By the time I arrived home, generalized soreness covered my body like a hardening plaster cast. I tried to treat the pain by focusing the pulsatile sensation, but couldn't pinpoint the source. Directing the pulse to my right leg made it hurt, which destroyed my ability to concentrate, and whole-body circulation while lying on my back made me squirm. When I finally drifted off to sleep, the pain blinked in a dark void like the lights of a distant aircraft flying at night.

Around 3:00 AM I woke to urinate. Groaning, I moved stiffly to the bathroom, but after flushing and turning to walk out, I felt something like a rubber band snap in my lower body and instantly fell, seized by the most excruciating pain I have ever experienced. Every muscle in my right leg was locked in a cast-iron spasm that almost blacked me out. The surface of my thigh bubbled like a liquid coming to a boil. I crawled into the bedroom, pulled myself up, and struggled through gritted teeth and groans to dress myself. Somehow I made it to my car and drove to an emergency room that was only minutes away.

An hour passed before I saw a doctor, the first I had seen in over a decade. He looked like a high school kid. After asking me about my symptoms, he said I had "sciatica," then disappeared from the exam room. Ten minutes later, an older neurologist appeared and had me lie supine on a table and do a few leg lifts. He disputed the younger doctor's diagnosis, advised me to lay off my exercise routine, and discharged me with a single Percocet that did absolutely nothing to relieve the pain.

Once back home, I dragged myself around the room for several minutes trying to find a posture that would relieve cramping that felt as though the muscles of my right thigh and pelvis were pulling my hip joint out of socket. The only way I could make the cramps let up even slightly was to sit on the edge of a table and hunch my back like that of a vulture perched on a tree branch. But within minutes pain emanated somewhere out of my lower body and sent my muscles into convulsion again. I dropped to floor and crawled like a poisoned bug to a couch where I twisted and turned until I found a position that gave some relief, which lasted no more than a couple of minutes. I stared at a window and watched it go from pitch black to pale light. In the pit of my stomach, I knew my life had changed forever, but I told myself I would heal through "the pulse."

After a day of more of the same, I went to a general practitioner, who repeated many of the same tests the emergency doctors had performed. He prescribed a horse-sized ibuprofen pill and counseled a wait-and-see approach that was standard protocol of the 1990's. I shut down the school for two weeks, which gave me enough time to progress from the stooped position of a monkey to standing for brief periods, but after only a few minutes, sometimes less than thirty seconds, the pain in my right hip and leg would force me to sit or lie down. Sleep was impossible. The pain roused me every half hour or so, and after another half hour of massaging and pulsing cramped muscles, I would drift off but then wake again to repeat the process. A month passed. Daily physical therapy, exhaustive Internet research, the horse-sized ibuprofen pills, and constantly "pulsing" the area seemed to bring some improvement. But then one day, while standing in the shower and moving my head to one side, the pain shifted from my right to left upper leg. There was now little question in my mind that I had ruptured a lumbar disc, a condition that had proven treatable with surgery only a third of the time.

As it turned out, my discs weren't the problem. My lumbar spine had snapped in two at a weak point in the vertebral facets, wing-shaped bones that run up and down the spine and form a kind of tree that holds in place the vertebrae and the discs sandwiched in between to cushion the vertebrae. The one I broke is called the pars interarticularis, a facet that acts as both hinge and support for the fourth and fifth lumbar vertebra. It would take eight years from the day of the injury before I would get a final diagnosis that I had a "pars defect," a genetic weakness in this area of the spine, which made wushu just about the worst kind of exercise I could do. When the pars facet snapped in two, the fourth lumbar vertebra slipped off of its disc cushion, a condition known as "spondylolisthesis." The slippage was initially forward and to the right, pinching major nerves within the spinal canal that controlled the right-side hip and leg muscles. The pinched nerves kept firing, causing the muscles to remain in a state of constant contraction. In such a state, muscles eventually fatigue and atrophy, which then leads to further orthopedic deterioration.

Illustration 34: Pars Defect and Spondylolisthesis

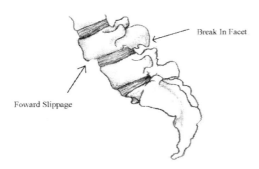

That is precisely what happened in my case, but with what I would define eventually as the RfR I was able to fight the deterioration so that I seesawed back and forth between being crippled and functional on an almost daily basis. Occasionally I felt almost normal, but then I would move the wrong way or strain too much in a certain direction and suffer through days of debilitating hip and leg pain that became increasingly bilateral. The worst times were at night, when between a couple of hours of sleep at a time I directed the RfR to dissipate the pain. X-rays and MRI's ordered by general practitioners and several neurologists revealed only a "slight scoliosis" (curvature) in my lumbar spine and a few bulging discs, but nothing appeared to have ruptured. After five years of living with this vacillating misery, I consulted an orthopedist, whose preliminary diagnosis was that I probably had hip arthritis, but after examining the x-rays the radiologist downplayed the possibility. Without images that showed serious damage that matched the pain I described, no physician was willing to advise anything more than for me to balance rest with reasonable activity, and when things got bad, to lay off wushu and any other vigorous sport, take ibuprofen, and do physical therapy that targeted weak muscles. In the meantime, my lower body remained in a constant state of inflammation, and my stress levels soared.

The smart thing to have done would have been to quit and go back to being a college professor. But then my sense that I had a genuine mission to fulfill got a big boost. A prominent publisher accepted a book I had finished writing about two years before my back injury. The book was a highly selective memoire of my two years in China that also introduced and taught aspects of Three Emperors Qigong. When the book came out, it caught the attention of China's Ministry of Sport and the BWI, which put me in the middle of a series of international efforts to combine Chinese and Western medical approaches that led to the formulation of RE, which four years later became the center of a second book that opened up the possibility of serious medical research that has led here to A^uI.

Meeting with China's Minister of Sport Wu Shaozu January 1999

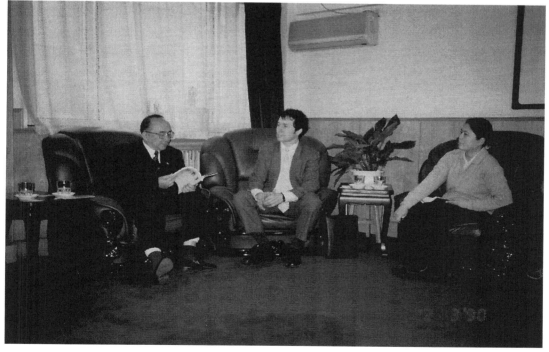

All the while, there were children to raise, an ex-wife to please and tussle with, a new relationship that became a marriage to serve, and a business to maintain. With my pride in the RfR and ability to use it to keep my pain under control, I couldn't abandon

148

what appeared to be increasing progress in exchange for returning to a profession that rarely tolerated more than a year's hiatus. In the meantime, like a leaky rowboat that takes on more water than can be bailed out, my lower-body filled up with pain that made me walk with a noticeable limp that brought concerned stares from the people around me. Occasionally my legs would buckle in mid-stride. No standing, sitting, or reclining position could make the pain stop. I became increasingly stiff to the point of being fully crippled.

Desperate and resigned, I turned to an internationally renowned spinal neurosurgeon, who took a series of more sophisticated MRI's that revealed the bad news. My pain was being caused by spinal stenosis—a narrowing of the interior of the spinal column—most probably caused by repeated fracturing of the pars interarticularis and subsequent spondylolisthesis. Without the support of an intact facet bone, the extreme activity I had been engaged in made the fourth and fifth lumbar vertebrae slip continuously, pinching nerves and generating constant inflammation. This, in turn, caused the lower spinal column to fill with scar tissue. He said the fracture apparently had fused into place, creating the appearance of the "mild scoliosis" the previous doctors had thought was no big deal. The stenosis was especially bad, he said, something he would expect to see in a ninety-year-old man. He recommended a "laminectomy," a procedure that would remove the "lamina"—a specific region of the outer posterior of the vertebra—and the spinal processes—the bones that visibly protrude and make the signature bumps of the backbone. Paring away these bony parts would release the nerves that were being pinched within the spinal column. But the procedure would destabilize the area once again, and so he also would have to perform a spinal fusion by inserting titanium screws on either side of the surgically altered lumbar. He conceded that the odds in general were not that great for back surgery, but someone of my age and fitness level had an excellent chance of making a decent recovery. Opening a copy of my second book I had brought with me, I pointed to photographs of stretches that put a great deal of stress on the lower back and asked if he thought I would be able to do any of them. He said yes. I tried to remember what it once felt like to move at full tilt without pain, and then said, "Let's do it." The surgeon nodded and told his assistant to schedule the surgery.

It took six hours. When I woke up in a hospital bed, the neurosurgeon, flanked on either side by a team of medical students who had observed and probably taken part in the operation, assured me that I would make a complete recovery, but I didn't. Instead I

First Back Surgery

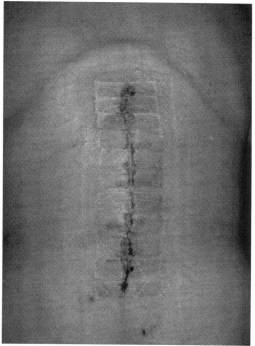

experienced an immediate series of debilitating setbacks. The first happened a few days after leaving the hospital, when I tried to walk around my neighborhood, what I had been told was an important aspect of my therapy. After less than a hundred yards, a suffocating malaise came over me, and terrible pain emanated from deep in my lower back, where a foot-long incision ran, held together by metal staples. Lurching from fences, parked cars, and trees for support, I got home, took off my shirt, and in the mirror saw that my back resembled water balloon about to burst. I spent the rest of the day lying on a chemical icepack and passing in and out of drug-induced sleep. A trip back to the neurosurgeon's office got me an audience with the neurosurgeon's assistant, who informed me that I never should have tried to walk around the block.

Two months passed and I still didn't seem to be making much progress. The physical therapist, who had had five surgeries on his own lumbar spine, was puzzled over why my muscles remained so tight, but insisted that I keep trying his prescribed exercises. The worst of these involved bringing my knee to my chest, the very thing that had brought on the first symptoms of the injury. One day, while straining to perform this exercise, I felt a bursting sensation in my lower back, and the familiar arresting pain poured lava-like down into my hips and legs.

Another trip back to the neurosurgeon resulted in my having to undergo a "myleogram," a nightmarish procedure that had me lying prone on a table while a foot-long needle was inserted directly into the site of the surgery in order to inject radioactive dye that would allow for a detailed x-ray of the interior of the spinal canal. It was supposed to be a five-minute job, but ended up taking about forty-five minutes because every time the boy-faced doctor tried to insert the needle, my body reflexively came off the table in a convulsion of pain beyond anything I had ever felt. It was as though I were being cut open without anesthesia. Finally, a more experienced physician appeared. Sticking his masked face down into mine, he told me it was going to hurt and that I should just hold it in. I gripped the sides of the table and felt the needle jab into my low back, followed by several jerky thrusts that were so forceful and quick my body didn't have time to rise up in rebellion.

The myleogram revealed that I had "adjacent disc disease," a common side effect in spinal fusion that demonstrates the ubiquity of the law of spiraling consequences of external problem solving. When I mentioned that not one of my pre-surgery consultations included the possibility of "adjacent disc disease," the neurosurgeon threw the blame back onto to me by suggesting I had "overdone it." Before I could respond, he stalked irritably out of the room, leaving me alone to wonder what was happening to me.

Filled with impotent rage to go along with renewed pain, I turned to a younger neurosurgeon who had a reputation for cleaning up messes caused by his more famous senior colleague. He confirmed the diagnosis that the disc just above the original pars fracture had herniated and was impinging on nerves to my right leg. He recommended another partial laminectomy, but then whipped out another x-ray, stuck it on the luminous screen, and explained that it looked to him that I might also have some arthritis in my hips that likely was adding to my problems. My heart sank as I explained with false confidence that my hips had been examined, x-rayed, and cleared by another specialist prior to my original spondylolisthesis diagnosis. He must have seen the disappointment on my face, because he looked down and said he was going to refer me to a hip specialist. I fell silent, staring at the luminous pictures of my skeleton.

The following day I was in the examination room of an orthopedic clinic facing another doctor, who took one look at the x-rays of my hips and said that I definitely needed hip replacement surgery. This time my heart went up into my throat, and I reiterated the earlier diagnosis I had gotten. From a folder he was carrying, he pulled out old x-rays and said that they were of lousy quality but showed pretty much the same thing as his x-rays.

"How much worse could it be?" I asked. "Those were taken just a little over a year ago."

"It's worse," he said. "I have no doubt that you need hip replacements."

I dropped my head to hide the moisture welling in my eyes and said, "I'll have to be crawling on the ground first."

The doctor shrugged, handed me a couple of brochures, and said bluntly that he would give me less than a year before I would be back.

Fuck you, I thought, as I walked out and struggled to get my legs in the car. On the drive home, I blasted my lower back and legs with the RfR. The pain dissolved until I got home and started walking again. I dragged myself up the stairs, lay on the bed, and opened one of the brochures to see an image of the procedure, which effectively involved amputating the leg from the femur head to mid-thigh and replacing the bone with a metal prosthesis. I pulled a pillow over my head and screamed as loud as I could.

Chapter 14

A Calculus of Death

As it turned out, the orthopedist and I made correct forecasts. After a little over a year that could serve as model for Hell, I was practically crawling when I went back to have the surgery.

This was preceded by several months of sleeplessness because of a deep, relentless ache that would wake me around 2:00 AM every night, starting vaguely in my lower back, and then extending sharply into my lower abdomen and down my right-side inner thigh to my kneecap, which felt as though it were slowly being pulled away from the bone. I was too exhausted to use the RfR. Shifting positions and distending abdominal muscles as much as possible were tricks that sometimes worked during the day, but had no effect at night. Crawling from the bed to lie face down on the floor and then bending my knee and bringing my right foot toward my butt stretched the great knot that ran from my kneecap up into my thigh and pelvis, but relief lasted only about thirty seconds. After a half hour or so of this, I would struggle to my feet and make my way down the stairs, the whole time fighting back the urge to sob for fear of waking my family. Once out of their earshot, I would burst into hysteria, begging God over and over to make the pain stop—the kind things someone might say under relentless, sadistic torture. For the next hour, I would use furniture, walls, and countertops to move back and forth between the kitchen sink and a thera-ball that sat in the den. From time to time, I would pause at the sink, grip the edge, and stand on my left leg while the right leg dangled like a deboned piece of meat, bent at the knee to keep it off the floor. On the thera-ball I would lie face down and roll forward until I was bent backward with my feet in the air, sobbing and begging God for mercy the entire time. As the windows facing east slowly began to glow, so too did the desire to escape from my pain by dying.

Over the course of three months of this torture, pleasure of even the smallest degree became impossible. My appetite vanished, and I lost twenty pounds, the lower half of my body shriveled-looking and cocked to the left in response to the right-side pain. Natural beauty, good memories, and proud accomplishments lost their power to soothe or even distract. All desire for human contact dried up, except for a hardened reflex to care for my wife and children. On more than one occasion, the thought of them was the only thing that stopped me from taking a headlong dive out of a window of the third story of my house.

That remnant of devotion to my family enabled me to take on the exhausting job of maintaining the few aspects of normal life I could manage. I climbed stairs by creative contortion, side-bending to the right, so that I could raise my left leg in a semi-normal fashion onto the first step. Then gripping handrails or pressing into walls, I would lean onto my left leg, still side-bent to the right, and swing my locked right leg up onto the step. For negotiating movement across flat surfaces, I used crutches. Driving a car entailed pushing the seat all the way back and sitting high up on a makeshift stack of blankets and pillows. This allowed me to lean into my right side and extend my eternally cramped right leg in order to operate the accelerator and brake. All paperwork had to be handled by using a clipboard while leaning back on the edge of a desk like a water-skier being pulled up by a speed boat.

I lasted another three months before scheduling the partial laminectomy, hoping to get enough relief from that seemingly less-severe procedure to buy a little more time. By then, the pain was so bad that I couldn't lie still long enough for the technicians to do a pre-operative MRI. They settled for a CAT scan, which took less than thirty seconds. I had to wait another two weeks for the surgery, and until then, I was not allowed any medication. I simply had to grin and bear it. During those two weeks, I slept only about one hour during the day and between one and two hours at night. The rest of the time I alternated between lying on each side and blasting my hips and legs with the RfR. My face looked sunken, eyes wizened and ringed with bruise-like circles. I ate only one small meal a day. By the time the day of the surgery finally came around, I longed to go to sleep and never wake up. When I arrived at the hospital intake room, I was such a disturbing sight that the nurses admitted me right away so that I didn't spook the other patients and their families, who stared with a mixture of horror and pity. Once in bed, feeling the cold infusion of an IV flowing into my arm, I lay on my side and tried to watch television. A middle-aged nurse with cat-eye glasses popped her shower-capped head through the curtain and asked how I was doing. I said not so well.

"I can help," she said. "I'm a certified Reiki healer."

Reiki is a Japanese version of "projected skill," as widely rejected in Japan as it is accepted and practiced among alternative healthcare practitioners in the West. Through a supposedly egoless state of consciousness, the Reiki practitioner can channel the healing power of "The Universe" through the body and project that power out of the hands into the passive sufferer. Beaten down too far to explain that I knew better, I smiled weakly and said, "Sure."

The nurse crouched beside the bed and closed her eyes like Dorothy in the *Wizard of Oz* before she says, "There's no place like home" and clicks together the heels of her ruby slippers. The nurse laid her hands on my lower back and concentrated. I didn't resist, letting myself go with the possibility that she could help me. All I felt was the mild warmth of the nurse's hands.

"There," she said, standing up and smiling. "Feel better?"

"Yes," I lied. "I believe I do."

The nurse beamed with satisfaction.

"Glad I could help."

She disappeared behind the curtain, which immediately opened again to reveal the comforting sight of an anesthesiologist, a young man very much at home in his white lab coat and conservative tie.

"Give me the drugs," I said.

He gave a tight, insincere smile and injected a narcotic into my IV. Within seconds I began drifting away from my pain, as though I had taken off in an airplane and was feeling momentary relief from the familiar earthward tug of gravity.

When I came to, I was in a recovery ward filled with empty beds, the fluorescence so bright it hurt. Then I realized the pain wasn't caused by the lights but by cramps emanating from the usual places on my right side. It was so intense I began shaking violently, as though I were being throttled.

"Make it stop!" I shouted hoarsely.

A nurse standing beside me was scribbling something on a chart. She was much younger than the Reiki master and her face was all business.

"Make it stop!" I repeated.

"Make what stop, sir?"

"Pain!"

"Sir, just breathe, sir."

"I breathe all the time. It doesn't work."

"Sir, if you'll just breathe—"

I gripped her arm with a vibrating hand.

"*If…you…don't…shut…up…I…am…going…to…kill…you!*" I said.

She pulled free and said, "Did you hear that?" to someone on the other side of the room.

"Sir, calm down," said a man's voice, his face swimming into view. He was young, probably an intern.

"*Fuck…you,*" I said, continuing to shake so furiously that the bed rattled. "*I'm…in…pain.*"

"Sir, there's no call for that kind of language."

"*Fuck…you,*" I repeated.

The nurse and the intern walked away, and then there was a slightly older woman stroking my arm and saying that she was there to help.

"I'm giving you more pain medicine now," she said.

I looked up from what seemed the bottom of a swimming pool, the woman's face a quivering, liquid mirage that faded into blackness.

I awoke in another ward and raised my head and saw across the room my neurosurgeon, towering over his cap-and-gown-covered medical team. The woman who had administered relief stood beside the surgeon. When she noticed I was awake, she came over, leaned down, and whispered in my ear that she had given me the most pain medication she had ever had to give a patient. I moved my right leg around in search of a remnant of the pain that had been eating me alive for months. It was still there but greatly reduced. I drifted off again into welcome drug-soaked oblivion and the fuzzy hope that I would wake again to feeling even better.

When I came too, the constriction in my right leg seemed to have stopped. The neurosurgeon explained that once he cut me open, he removed a swollen ligament that sat right on the nerve, causing the muscles of my lower right side to contract. He qualified this good report with warning that some of my pain might not be gone because I had "other issues." At the time I was feeling too good to register much of anything else.

After release from the hospital, I tried to stay focused on the apparent good the surgery had done for my right leg, but I still moved stiffly and had to take small steps. Going upstairs or even a slight incline was also difficult and quickly became painful to the point where I could not lift my right leg to the height of a street curb. A short time later I had to avoid all stairs, except those at home, which I continued negotiating by creative contortion. Every day I stared out the window with bitter longing at runners bounding along the streets of our neighborhood. Even the sight of elderly men and women walking their dogs filled me with envy. A few months post-surgery, I experienced a final-straw moment after driving to town to take care of some paperwork. The walking distance between my handicapped parking space and the office building entrance was about one hundred yards. I checked my watch and started hobbling. People continually passed by, moving at clips I would have given several fingers, perhaps an arm, to manage. I finally made it to the door, leaned exhaustedly against the wall, and looked at my watch. It had taken me eight minutes. When I got home, I scheduled an appointment with the hip surgeon for the following day.

Pre-operative education was as depressing as it was enlightening. I was shown an x-ray of a healthy ball-and-socket hip joint: a well-defined head as smooth and round as a tennis ball that fit into a clear, curved space in the hip bone. In contrast, an x-ray of my hip joint showed no space between the ball and socket, as though the thigh and pelvis had been ground into one another, which is what happened on the left side. The right side was worse. The ball had been wrenched entirely out of the socket, making the right leg shorter than the other. I explained that when I felt my back snap the first time, it seemed as though the convulsing muscles were pulling my right hip out of joint. The hip surgeon shrugged and said it was possible, but that it was equally possible that I had simply been born with shallow hip sockets, another inherent condition that made wushu, especially some of the high kicking techniques the wrong form of exercise for me. I doubted this explanation because up until the injury I managed the highest of kicks with little or no fallout. I kept asking questions. Which came first, the back injury or the hips? If I had had the hips done first, could I have avoided back surgery? To each question the surgeon responded with non-answers, insisting there was no way to tell, but that now that baby boomers were aging orthopedists were seeing more and more hip-and-low back degenerative conditions, especially in jock-types like myself. That was why he felt so encouraged by the development of new metal-on-metal artificial hips that were taking the place of the traditional ceramic-on-ceramic or metal-on-plastic prostheses that usually lasted no longer than ten years before they needed to be replaced. According to the surgeon, the total metal hip replacements would outlast the life of the recipient, who also would enjoy greater athletic ability.

I was sold on the spot, and even agreed to have both hips replaced in a single surgery because the surgeon said it would save money and save me the misery of having to go through two separate recoveries. Before I left the office, I was asked whether or not I wanted to lay away blood for a transfusion that may be necessary during the surgery, a question that had not been asked of me before either of my back surgeries. I had read in the brochure that transfusions were necessary in only one percent of cases, so I declined. Considering what had been happening to me for the past decade, I should have known that somehow I would end up landing in the unlucky one percentile.

The three months of time that led up to my hip surgery was like one non-stop brawl with my pain. The severe degenerative condition of my hips had so inflamed and tightened the muscles of my thighs, hips, and abdominals that my torso was pulled forward into a stooped position that in turn strained and torn down my lower back. I spent most of my time downstairs, blasting my back and hips with the RfR while lying on a day bed. Getting up for any reason was an ordeal. The few purposeful tasks I had been clinging to, such as preparing meals and washing dishes, were out of the question. I was finally a total invalid that had to be waited on. My wife took up the task, but her own misery grew noticeably every day. A kind of detached despair I hadn't experienced before came over me, a deep recognition that all my concerns, drives, and desires were self-manufactured illusions that were about to end. An odd certainty that I was not going to survive this third surgery nested comfortably in my thoughts. On the day the anesthesiologist and nurses rolled me down the hall for the operation, I was at peace with the knowledge that I was either going to die in surgery or emerge crippled for the rest of what would be a short life that I was now willing to relinquish.

When I awoke from anesthesia, I felt the most rested I had been in years, though I knew that if I tried moving my legs, which were being electronically kneaded by ankle-to-hip leggings, my good mood would shift. My wife, who seemed to have been crying, and the surgical team were in the room. My wife started talking to me about being still a little swollen from all the fluids they had pumped into me. Apparently I had been in an induced coma on a ventilator.

"What happened?" I said cheerfully.

She deferred to the hip surgeon, who said they were still doing tests to see if there was something in one of the units of blood he had to give me.

"Blood?" I said.

Laying a hand on my shoulder, he said he had never seen anything like it. He started describing some sort of problem that I listened to without fully understanding, but over the course of the next couple of days I was able to construct a narrative of what had apparently gone wrong. The surgeon had started on the left hip, because it was the more pathological of the two, and in the process I lost somewhere in the neighborhood of four pints of blood, which was a little extreme, so the surgeon hesitated about replacing the right hip. But because he felt it needed to be done in order for me to make an optimal recovery, he gave the go-ahead. They flipped me over onto my left side, but as soon as they cut into my right hip, blood began welling so profusely that they thought they had accidentally severed a major blood vessel. While they scrambled to find the cut vein or artery, my blood pressure dropped to near nothing and my heart stopped. They responded with a blast of epinephrine and a massive infusion of plasma and fluids. By the time they had me stable, my entire blood supply had been replaced. The conclusion was that I belonged to another outlier category of persons born with an overabundance of capillaries in my hip bones. I decided not to share the speculation that directing the RfR to that region of the body for so long and with such frequency was probably what did it. No one would have believed me.

After a week of bed rest and physical therapy, I was ready to go home, much to the surprise of the physicians in charge, especially given that I had two hip replacements and had nearly bled to death. Once at home, I got around using a walker. After another week I was able to go to two canes. A few days later, I dropped one of the canes. A few days after that, I was able to walk without assistance. For the first time in years, I could take the stairs without horrible pain or contorting my body. In addition to the physical therapy exercises I had been assigned, I practiced Taijiquan several times a day, using whole-body circulation of the RfR to dampen the pro-inflammatory molecules that still saturated my blood stream. Carefully and assiduously working toward greater flexibility, I felt the pain, tightness, and frailty of having my legs cut open and sawed off at mid-femur give way to a sense of strength and looseness. The only worrisome signs were a loss of sensation in my left big toe that had been with me since my first back surgery and a new numbness that spread across my right shin like a sock. According to my surgeon, these were probably irreversible consequences I would simply have to live with.

Two months after hip surgery, I could run a mile in about nine minutes. A few months later I managed three miles, averaging a little over seven minutes per mile. It hurt, most pointedly in my knees, because my hip joints were so strong that the impact registered in the next link in the lower body's system of musculoskeletal shock absorbers. My back didn't exactly feel great either, the muscles in my right hip, abdomen, and back locking in a protective embrace around my damaged lumbar spine. But my vast experience with pain told me the problem would pass, so long as I exercised with caution and proper self-maintenance.

Shortly thereafter I started swimming at an outdoor pool in a public park beside our neighborhood. I expected to restore cardiovascular fitness as quickly as I had after previous surgeries, but I was wrong. I could barely swim two lengths before having to stop, my entire upper body a knot of vexed muscle. My heart seemed about to explode in my chest, and I clung to the wall gasping for air as though I had never before swum laps. By comparison my legs felt fine. Concerned that my near-death experience on the operating table had somehow robbed me of the vagal tone that had made the RfR so wonderfully effective for me over the years, I consulted my surgeon. He assured me that temporary loss of cardiovascular fitness was common in cases like mine. It would come back, he said.

A month later it did come back, and I was able to swim my usual workouts with less trouble than I experienced prior to my first surgery. It was as though I had been reborn, a sense I amplified by following each swim with stretching, Taijiquan, and whole-body circulation of the RfR. I did this beside a small pond, surrounded by hardwoods and willows, similar to what I had enjoyed when I practiced in the Imperial Garden of Beijing.

Though I reveled in my resurrected ability to enjoy movement and the quiet beauty of my new practice setting, I turned my attention increasingly inward, concerned that the blood with which I had been transfused was rife with unknown micro-contaminants. I concentrated deeply on back-to-front circulation of the RfR. With each session, the inside of my head swelled and roiled like a snake rousted from hibernation, an internal resistance to the RfR that felt similar to trying to hold a high-pressure hose pipe underwater. Welts and boils began popping out on my skin and scalp. The lymph nodes in my left armpit swelled and my entire left arm ached as though the muscles had been strained. After about a month, these symptoms subsided, the RfR flowed smoothly, and I was able to let my attention drift outward again.

Sitting on a bench, bathed in the cool pall of wind and moisture blowing off the pond, I circulated the RfR like a whole-body hymn of praise and gratitude to feel at home in my body and the world. Frogs croaked and rustled the reeds of the shoreline, and dragonflies careened through the dappled air, devouring flies and mosquitoes that would have ruined my meditation. Occasionally a fish startled the water to snap at a low-flying dragonfly, and when I cracked an eye to investigate I spied the tiny head of a turtle sculling slowly before dropping back beneath the pond's surface.

The image took me back to a central metaphor in my first book that used swimming on-versus-under the water's surface to explain the difference between Western exercise and Far Eastern mind-body meditation. Western athletes and even athletic martial artists were like surface swimmers, making lots of waves and putting on a spectacle. The underwater swimming of East Indian yogis and Qigong masters was invisible to the naked eye but revealed depths of reality beyond the comprehension of surface dwellers.

At the time I wrote that, I believed Far Eastern mind-body practices penetrated the truth as deeply as possible. But now I know the deeper truth that pain and suffering breaks down the illusory world until all that remains to surrender is pulsatile. Beyond that limit, we can only imagine what happens. Perhaps the pulsatile self becomes lost in the orchestral vibrations that fill the background of the physical universe. Or it may ride off on some oscillating frequency into other worlds that sit beside this one, invisible to us but resonant with our pulsatile nature. And while we wait on this side of our final limit, the illusory self glides along on the wave that is our deepest source of life, vacillating between hope and surrender as our circumstances shift between favor and punishment. We cannot help but react this way, because beneath our transient layers a waveform is what we are, until the final moment arrives and we *are* no more.

Epilogue

In 2010, the FDA declared certain kinds of metal-on-metal hip implants unsafe because of a growing number of complaints of side effects and outright failures that were causing recipients to undergo revision surgery. The manufacturers recalled their prostheses, including the kind implanted in me. Doctors were told to re-examine all their patients for signs of trouble. The news media reported impending lawsuits that promised billions in retribution. Law firms started trolling for clients by running advertisements high and low, from *The New York Times* to primetime commercial television.

My surgeon had implanted the recalled hip joint only on the left side. He had wanted to do both, because the ball-and-socket was larger, allowing for a more robust range of motion. But the greater size meant he had to shave away more bone to place the metal socket into the biological one, and the concavity of my right socket had deteriorated too badly for the design to work. This was the one silver lining in this dark cloud of bad news, which partly explained why my left hip had never felt as good as my right. But this go-round perhaps I would be one of the lucky ones because my level of function and general absence of pain was so much better. My surgeon ordered x-rays and said things looked fine, but just to be sure he had my blood tested for metal contamination. A few days later I got an alarming call from his assistant saying I needed to come in immediately because the metal levels in my blood were hundreds of time higher than what was considered safe. An MRI showed that the discomfort I had been feeling in my left hip had an actual cause: a fluid mass, or pseudo-tumor, on the outside of my hip, in the soft tissue adjacent to where the ball met the socket. Apparently the action of the metal parts moving against one another continuously shaved off micro-particles that accumulated near the implant and provoked a pro-inflammatory response.

I took the news with a surprising lack of emotion, a gift of the suffering I had been through the previous twelve years. The worst case scenario was that I wouldn't make it through revision surgery and shortly thereafter and my wife and children would get millions in a wrongful death settlement. Second worst case I would come out of the surgery crippled, another consequence that likely would result in considerable compensation. But there was also the possibility that I could self-treat my metal poisoning and soft-tissue inflammatory build-up with the RfR and selective methods along the $A''I$ spectrum. I had nothing to lose by trying.

For insurance, I contacted a high-powered law firm that was eager to have me as a client because of the astronomically high metal levels in my blood—the highest they had seen in the thousands of cases they had reviewed. They assured that a big settlement was due me. All I had to do was to have the revision surgery and join the first wave of plaintiffs scheduled to go up against the manufacturer. It seemed like sound advice, but once I had gotten the bad news, I had focused the RfR assiduously on the area where the MRI had shown the fluid mass and the pain and discomfort had greatly diminished. I also stopped running and performing the more challenging wushu routines I had taken out of mothballs, turning instead almost exclusively to swimming, calisthenics, biking, Taijiquan, and less-demanding wushu that didn't overtax the muscles of the lower body. A few months later I went back to have my blood re-analyzed, and the metal levels had dropped considerably.

As I dug into the medical science on metal contamination, I discovered that the evidence of damage to health had come from those who mined the metals and in the process inhaled massive amounts of metallic particulates. While miners suffered a raft of illnesses that ranged from cognitive breakdown to cancer, there really wasn't any hard evidence that kind of metal residue I had would cause those kinds of health problems. In fact, the metals had a reasonable half-life and theoretically were being expelled through all the body's excretory systems.

As the lawsuits evolved, estimates of the total cost for the manufacturers of the faulty device were in the neighborhood of nine billion. These numbers sparked a series of investigative reports that dug into the ugly reality of the U.S. healthcare system's runaway costs, driven by expensive procedures like hip replacement surgeries for a growing elderly population served largely by Medicare. Ironically, my own malingering at the fourth meta-$A''I$ level had made me both beneficiary and part of the rising healthcare cost problem decried at the outset of this book. But I also walk my own talk. I decided against getting my left hip revised, despite warnings from my lawyers that without doing so I stood little or no chance of my recovering any money in a settlement with the manufacturer. I didn't make this decision lightly. Second and third opinions from top-tier hip specialists confirmed that while the metal levels in my blood were concerning, immediate revision was unwarranted because I had such high functionality and relatively tolerable symptoms of actual harm. Naturally all were skeptical of my claims to be able to manage the inevitable side effects of the external re-engineering of my locomotion system. But because of the RfR and all the advantages of having advanced $A''I$, I remain hopeful with good cause.

Since the 2010 metal-on-metal hip recall, my situation has changed very little. I still have a fluid mass on my left hip that occasionally causes pain if I overdo it. But my physical prowess in the water and range of motion in my lower back and legs has never been better. At this point, I see no compelling reason to doubt that practicing *unified fitness* will enable me to heed my own counsel in this book, even in a compromised state. Data, theory, and experience indicate that cultivating the pulsatile self through the RfR not only gives the ability to sense and direct the autonomic cardiovascular and immune systems to self-treat symptoms, but also can help to expel contaminants from my blood, along with all the other inflammation caused by constant infection and stress. I take great comfort in these supportable claims, but the limits of the pulsatile self and the hazards of imagination are never far from my thoughts.

Works Cited

Chase, Nancy L., et al. "Research Swimming and All-Cause Mortality Risk Compared With Running, Walking, and Sedentary Habits in Men." *International Journal of Aquatic Research and Education.* 2.3 (Aug 2008). n.pag. Web. 31 Dec. 2015.

Chiesa A, and A. Serretti. A Systematic Review of Neurobiological and Clinical Features of Mindfulness Meditations. *Psychological Medicine* 40.8 (Aug 2010) 1239-52. Web. 31 Dec. 2015.

Davalos, Albert R., et al. "Senescent cells as a source of inflammatory factors for tumor progression." *Cancer Metastasis Review.* 2010 Jun; 29(2): 273–283. (Apr 13 2010) Web. 31 Dec. 2015.

Dusek, J. A., and Herbert Benson. "Mind-body Medicine: a Model of the Comparative Clinical Impact of the Acute Stress and Relaxation Responses." *Minnesota Medicine* 92.5 (May 2009): 47-50. Print.

Haenzel, A., et al. "The Relationship between Heart Rate Variability and Inflammatory Markers in Cardiovascular Diseases. *Psychoneuroendocrinology* 33.1305 (2008): n.pag. Web. 31 Dec. 2015.

Hall, Kathryn T., et al. "Catechol-O-Methyltransferase val158met Polymorphism Predicts Placebo Effect in Irritable Bowel Syndrome." *PLoS ONE* 7.10 (Oct 23 2012) n.pag. Web. 31 Dec. 2015.

Hölzel, Britta K., et al. "Mindfulness Practice Leads to Increases in Regional Brain Gray Matter Density." *Psychiatry Research Neuroimaging.* 191.1 (Jan 30 2011) 36–43. Web 31 January 2016.

Liu, Haisheng, et al. "Olfactory Route for Cerebrospinal Fluid Drainage into the Cervical Lymphatic System in a Rabbit Experimental Model. *" Neural Regeneration Research.* 7.10 (Apr 5 2012) 766–771. Web. 31 Dec. 2015.

Louveau, Antoine, et al. "Structural and Functional Features of Central Nervous System Lymphatic Vessels." *Nature.* 523.7560 (2015) 337-341. Web. 31 Dec. 2015.

McCauliff, Kathleen. "How Your Cat Is Making You Crazy." *The Atlantic Monthly.* March 2012. n.pag. Web. 31 Dec. 2015.

Ornish D., et al. "Changes in Prostate Gene Expression in Men Undergoing an Intensive
Nutrition and Lifestyle Intervention. *Proceedings of the National Academy of
Science U SA*. 105.24 (June 17 2008): 8369-74. Print.

Peng, C-K, et al. Exaggerated Heart Rate Oscillations during Two Meditation
Techniques. *International Journal of Cardiology*. 70 (1999), 101-107.

Pinto, A, et.al. "Effects of Physical Exercise on Inflammatory Markers of Atherosclerosis."
Current Pharmaceutical Design. 18.28 (2012) 4326-49.

Pert, Candice. *The Molecules of Emotion*. New York: Touchstone, 1999. 162-164, Print.

Reynolds, Gretchen. "Exercise and the 'Good' Bugs in our Gut." *The New York Times*.
June 18, 2014 n.pag. Web 25 February 2016.

Rich, T., et al. "Assessment of Cardiovascular Parameters with the CareTaker Device
during Meditation." *The International Journal of Complementary and Alternative
Medicine*. (2016) 4(5):00135.

Rich, T., et al. "Assessment of Cardiovascular Parameters during Meditation with Mental
Targeting in Swimmers." *Evidence-based Complementary and Alternative
Medicine*. " (2016) Article ID 7923234, 5 pages, Web. 12 Feb. 2016.

Sandercock, G.R, et al. "Effects of Exercise on Heart Rate Variability: Inferences from
Meta-analysis." *Medicine and Science in Sports and Exercise*. 3.37 (March 2005)
433-9.

Sloan, R.P., et al. "Interval Variability Is Inversely Related to Inflammatory Markers: The
Cardia Study." *Molecular Medicine* 13.178 (2007): n.pag. Web. 31 Dec. 2015.

"Statistical Communiqué on the 2011 National Economic and Social Development."
National Bureau of Statistics of China. 2012. Web. 31 December 2015.

Tracey, Kevin. "The Inflammatory Reflex." *Nature*. 420 (Dec 19 2002) 853-859. Web. 31
Dec. 2015.

Wright, P.A., et al. "A Pilot Study of Qigong Practice and Upper Respiratory Illness in
Elite Swimmers." *American Journal of Chinese Medicine*: 3: 39 (2011) 461-475.
Web 31 December 2015.

Yost, T.L., and A. G. Taylor. "Qigong as a Novel Intervention for Service Members with Mild Traumatic Brain Injury. *Explore: Journal of Science and Healing* May-Jun. 3 (2013). 142-149. Web. 31 December 2015.

Zierath, J., et al. "Acute Exercise Remodels Promoter Methylation in Human Skeletal Muscle." *Cell Metabolism.* 15. 3 (March 2012). 405-411.

General Sources by Chapter

Chapter 10: Ewald, Paul W. *Plague Time*. New York: First Touchstone Edition, 1999.

Chapters 12, 13, and 14: Palmer, David. *Qigong Fever*. NY: Columbia University Press, 2007.

Chapters 13 and 14: Ownby, David. *Falun Gong and the Future of China*. NY: Oxford University Press, 2009.

Made in the USA
Coppell, TX
08 March 2021